PENGUIN BOOKS

HOW DID I BECOME MY PARENT'S PARENT?

Harriet Sarnoff Schiff is the author of two classic works on grieving, *The Bereaved Parent* and *Living Through Mourning*, as well as *How Did I Become My Parent's Parent?* and *The Support Group Manual*. All of her books are available from Penguin. A former reporter for *The Detroit News*, she has lectured throughout the United States, Canada, and Australia and appeared on television shows such as *Donahue*, *Oprah*, and the *Today* show. More recently, as the Corporate Admissions Coordinator for a group of thirteen nursing homes, she worked with admissions personnel and social workers and ran activity programs and support groups for residents and family members. She lives in Birmingham, Michigan.

How Did I Become My Parent's Parent?

Harriet Sarnoff Schiff

PENGUIN BOOKS

PENGUIN BOOKS
Published by the Penguin Group
Penguin Books USA Inc., 375 Hudson Street,
New York, New York 10014, U.S.A.
Penguin Books Ltd, 27 Wrights Lane, London W8 5TZ, England
Penguin Books Australia Ltd, Ringwood, Victoria, Australia
Penguin Books Canada Ltd, 10 Alcorn Avenue,
Toronto, Ontario, Canada M4V 3B2
Penguin Books (N.Z.) Ltd, 182–190 Wairau Road,
Auckland 10, New Zealand

Penguin Books Ltd, Registered Offices:
Harmondsworth, Middlesex, England

First published in the United States of America by
Viking Penguin, a division of Penguin Books USA Inc. 1996
Published in Penguin Books 1997

10 9 8 7 6 5 4 3 2 1

THE LIBRARY OF CONGRESS HAS CATALOGUED THE HARDCOVER AS FOLLOWS:
Schiff, Harriet Sarnoff.
How did I become my parent's parent?/Harriet Sarnoff Schiff.
p.   cm.
ISBN 0-670-85543-X (hc.)
ISBN 0 14 02.3714 3 (pbk.)
1. Aging parents—Care—United States.   2. Adult children—United States—
Attitudes.   3. Nursing homes—United States.   I. Title.
HQ1063.6.S35   1996
306.874—dc20   95–42010

Printed in the United States of America
Set in Garamond Light
Designed by Richard Oriolo

To the memory of
Irving Sarnoff
Mickie Ambrose
. . . and of course Robby

my father, my friend, and my son,
who will always be in my heart

Preface

◇

In the time since my intense focus on bereavement I have spent much time working with the families of elderly people.

My years as the corporate admissions coordinator for a group of thirteen nursing homes brought me in daily contact with those who were about to become residents and even more with those who had decided to place their mothers or fathers in one of the facilities.

While at first I assumed the life cycle of aging would be less pain-ridden than death I soon discovered my error. In the course of my work with families and the interviews I conducted for this book, I once again saw a great deal of pain and a great many tears.

When adult children find themselves in the impossible position of trying to function as their parents' parents they frequently suffer great emotional distress. They feel uneasy and indecisive. They wonder if there was not something more, something better, that they could have done.

These feelings of pain and the fear that they have done the wrong thing, or perhaps not done enough that was right, can be lessened when one knows others have experienced these issues and survived the hurt.

It is my hope this book will help people identify their own pain with the experiences shared herein. When you read about a family's situation that closely corresponds to what you are living with or have lived through, somehow your own distress is eased.

As this book will demonstrate, *you are not alone*.

Your drama is being played out in varying forms by countless others who share your difficulty.

Added to this is the gift of their shared solutions. Just seeing how someone else has dealt with a problem may offer you hope. You may see one part of how a family handled a circumstance and that may start your mind on an approach entirely different from the one you had considered. It may be your first step down a path you had never before contemplated.

Because the U.S. population is aging and the so-called Baby Boomers are now coping with elderly parents, the media and government are turning their attention to how we will handle the many complex issues that arise.

Transiency is a great factor in this era. How can adult children still be supportive to aging parents when all are separated by many miles? Surprisingly, there is much that can be done and you will see instances of how some families cope with this experience throughout the book.

While certainly this guidance will be useful to every adult who has aging parents, parents themselves may profit from reading this book. They may learn some wise ways of staying in the picture and being wanted and sought after by their children.

Not only will families find a new understanding, but those in the helping fields will also find comfort in knowing their guidance has proved valuable. I hope this book will be read by social workers, nursing home administrators, members of the clergy, funeral directors, home health care workers, administrators of Assisted Living apartments and senior citizen buildings, and those working in fields dealing with age-related illnesses such as Parkinson's disease, Alzheimer's disease, and heart conditions.

After speaking with many hundreds of people, I found it always came back to the fact that loss is loss.

I saw the familiar look of pain that I had come to know through my interviewing and lecturing. I saw apprehension in the eyes of many. Were they doing the loving thing? Would Mother be properly cared for?

While running support groups for these people I heard such questions crop up again and again.

Since working in this field I have learned that nursing homes, by and large, are not frightening or spooky places. Rather, good care is given by caring people most of the time.

As long as we convince ourselves we are sending our parents to some hell hole we will suffer a guilt that is usually unnecessary.

In a sense the reputation nursing homes have is no different from the reputation funeral directors had in an earlier time. Just as funeral directors are now being accepted as honored members of society, it is my hope the same will occur with nursing homes and administrators. We live in a world where many families require two incomes merely to survive. The need for a proper place to house an elderly parent is critical.

A nursing home is not the answer for everyone. There are many people of means who do not need this type of care. There are many excellent home health care agencies that can provide exceptional support to an ailing and aging parent. That is always the first choice if funds are available. But having to choose another alternative does not make any of us bad human beings.

For this book I have interviewed people from nearly every state in the union but I have made it a point to change names and other identifying characteristics of those whose stories I told. My promise of privacy gave me more information and insight into the intense feelings of those with whom I spoke.

Also, I did not wish to address issues particular to specific ethnic groups as I felt to do so would detract from my message of support and unity with all who experience this difficult circumstance. My goal, instead, was to bring you a work that you could relate to regardless of background.

Like *The Bereaved Parent*, this is a book about people.

It is my hope that you will even smile a little and feel an easing in your heart.

HARRIET SARNOFF SCHIFF

Acknowledgments

◈

Thanks are due to Dr. Ronald Trunsky, associate chairman, department of psychiatry, Sinai Hospital of Detroit, with a specialty in geropsychiatry; Susan Belaney, geriatric social worker, Oakland General Hospital; Doreen Lichtman, M.S.W., C.S.W., Botsford Hospital; Audrey Wasserman Chase, C.S.W., program supervisor, adult well-being services; Marlana J. Geha, Ph.D., specialist in working with the aged and their caregivers; Marilyn Gilbert, Ph.D., specialist in significant loss; Donald J. Bortz, for offering me the opportunity to serve; and Judy Smythe, my nursing home mentor, from whom I gathered invaluable information.

For their insights through the years I wish to also thank the social work staffs of these Michigan Hospitals: St. Joseph Hospital, Pontiac; Detroit Receiving Hospital; Beaumont Hospital, Royal Oak; Sinai Hospital, Detroit; Riverview Hospital, Detroit; Pontiac Osteopathic Hospital; Bi-County General Hospital, Warren; University of Michigan, Ann Arbor; Holy Cross Hospital, Detroit; The Parkinsons Foundation of Michigan; The Cancer Foundation of Michigan; and Catholic Social Services of Detroit. I sincerely appreciate your work with me, and the insights you shared so willingly.

On a personal note, I wish to thank some special people whom I dearly love. They are a strong part of my life and have been there through good times and bad: Dale, Sharon, Robyn, and Samantha Schiff; Stacie, Tom, and Jason Fine; Roz and Barry Rope and my terrific nephews; Eileen and Gordon Abel and their wonderful brood; Sandra and Larry Schiff and their terrific family; Pat Gorman, for years of friendship and support; Judy and Howard Koss and all their loved ones; Cheryl and Bob Dewitt and the people they hold dear; Noreen and John Zimmer and their special ones; Barbara and Paul Begun and all of those they treasure. And, of course, Ellen Levine, agent extraordinaire, who is always there for me!

To my editor, Caroline J. White, whose sensitivity to written work makes it impossible to know where I left off and she began: thank you, Caroline, for everything. I hope we are always a team.

Thank you all for your concern and caring and for being in my corner when I needed you.

Most of all, I thank my love of so many years, my husband, Sander. I cherish what we share together; it is beyond price or destruction. I love you and our love and our special friendship.

Contents

———◇———

HOW DID I
BECOME MY
PARENT'S PARENT?

INTRODUCTION:
A NEW ROLE

◈

From the moment we draw our first breath most of us are headed to that point in our lives when we will become Chadults. A Chadult is an adult whose parents are still living. "Chadult" is a contraction of "child-adult"—and sometimes that can be quite a contraction!

Most Chadults have reached that reasonably comfortable

stage in life where they know where they are heading and hope they will arrive at their destination intact.

They have a sense of purpose. Many have grown children who are in college or starting their own careers. Some Chadults have young grandchildren.

Being a Chadult is not about being a given age. It is instead about being at a certain time in one's life when one has a reasonable amount of freedom to live and play and travel and work.

Basically, it all sounds fairly comfortable . . . and for many it remains so. People of comfortable financial means can remain at their ease indefinitely. They can pay for and arrange for things to be smooth.

People whose parents remain self-sufficient or die quietly in their sleep one night can remain in this comfortable flow. There is no reason to think the flow will change.

This does not mean to imply that such Chadults lack love or caring or involvement. It merely means the resources needed, whether time or money, are readily at hand.

But most of us are not that easy in our Chadulthood where our parents are concerned. We start to feel tuggings and pullings that have become unfamiliar in our free and easy world.

The time may come when all that freedom and comfort is taken away. Not by our own choice, but by the circumstances with which we are faced when our parents age and perhaps become infirm. Sometimes Chadults make the mistake of thinking their parents want their help when they emphatically do not. Other times Chadults let their parents fumble along when they should intervene.

As children many of us played the game monkey in the middle. Most of us who remember it probably remember disliking it intensely! Oh, not when we were on the outside teasing, but when we were in the middle being the monkey trying to reach the ball.

This sensation, long forgotten by most of us, comes back like the memory of a toothache that would not quit. The feeling of being tugged in this direction and that, and the uneasiness, are profound when we are confronted with parents who need parenting.

But there are some questions that require answering. The primary one, of course, is who made the decision about intervention? If you, the Chadult, made it yourself, you may not have realized how deeply you would become involved. You may have volunteered to help Mom get resettled in a more comfortable situation. But did you ever dream you would be getting calls demanding rides here or there or everywhere?

If you had the decision thrust upon you, you may find the feeling of being trapped is very much that monkey-in-the-middle sensation. You know the tasks must be done, but a certain lovingness leaves you and is often replaced with resentment and all the other feelings of loss we experience as time goes on.

Perhaps by viewing these feelings and experiences with some dispassion and the certainty that you are not alone, you can go forward into this strange new world of role reversal and even see some humor along the way.

By the time a man realizes that his father was usually right, he has a son who thinks he's usually wrong!
—Anonymous

Chapter 1

IN THE

BEGINNING

◈

O nce three elderly mothers, all widowed, were enjoying lunch and boasting about their sons.

Mrs. Jones leaned casually forward and said, "My boy is so wonderful! Whenever the first sign of frost comes along he immediately calls the airline and a hotel in Florida and he makes a reservation for me to spend the winter there as his gift!"

Her two companions nodded and commented on his kindness.

But then Mrs. Smith told the women about her son. "He is the best young man. As soon as winter threatens he calls a real estate broker in Florida and rents a house for me at the beach. Imagine, my own private home!"

"Well, I really have to compliment you on your sons," said Mrs. Brown. "But let me tell you about mine. He loves me so much that every week he goes to a man and pays him two hundred dollars. And you know what for? Just so he can sit there and talk about *me!* His mother! Now *that's* a son!"

While certainly there is a delicious chuckle in this tale, it raises certain questions.

Among the most important: were the mothers consulted?

Certainly the intentions were the best, but would these same sons have made similar arrangements for their own adult children or their friends?

Most likely they would not. At the very least they would call to inquire about whether the plan was welcome, or if there were any major events on the other person's schedule.

What may appear to be kindness to one person may, to another, be perceived as high-handedness.

If Mother has trouble making decisions, are we being loving children by making them for her, or are we further diminishing her capacities?

After all, for many years Mother did the deciding. The initiating. The planning. What happens when a Chadult reverses the roles?

How frequently does this happen with people who have aging parents? How often has there been the automatic assumption—or presumption—that making decisions for parents does not necessarily require the input of the parent?

Remember, in the United States the government governs

with the *consent* of the governed. That is a fundamental right of the people. Have we taken this right away from our own parents?

Of course there is another important matter introduced by this story. Few of us have had idyllic childhoods. The son who spent his money at the psychiatrist's did not do so out of joy! There were probably many issues from his youth that needed resolving. Were his parents too lenient? Were they too strict? Did they demand too much? Did they ignore him? Was there another and more favored child?

These are not light issues. They are issues that many carry into adulthood. There may be a time during those special years when we are building lives for ourselves, with careers, marriages, and children of our own, when the old issues are put on a back burner. But when we become Chadults many of us shut down the back burner, and every hurt and slight is right at the front, burning and hurting us just as if we were once again children.

Many things begin to change slowly when Chadults believe it is necessary to take control.

Sometimes Mother or Father sends us early warning signals that things are beginning to change.

It can be something as small as an increased demand on the part of the parent to be called daily. This may be for the obvious reason—wanting attention. As parents age you must remember that many of their peers are dead. Their world becomes narrower and narrower and the attention of their children becomes, in the parent's mind, essential.

Because many women of this generation were not part of the great move to "find themselves" or in some other way to be liberated, many mothers who are alone are indeed dependent. Many do not drive. As more and more people create a suburbanized environment for themselves they are losing things that once were taken for granted. Walking to the corner and hopping on the local bus may be a thing of the past.

Today, if an elderly person who does not drive wants to go somewhere she must call a Chadult or a neighbor, or if she is truly fortunate there might be a suburban bus that will come to her home and take her to her destination.

But the real problem is the complete lack of preparedness for their new situation which most aging parents have to face. They simply have not thought about the what-ifs. Many of them still feel so young in spirit that preparedness is something for others, not *them*. Unfortunately our bodies and our spirit do not remain synchronized as the aging process goes inexorably forward.

Rebecca who is well into her eighties continued to insist on having big holiday dinners at her home. Her daughter had begged her to stop and offered to have them in her own home. Rebecca was adamant. She was doing the dinner.

This, on the face of it, sounds admirable. To outsiders the "old lady" sounds full of moxie! Most often that is only the surface picture.

To accomplish this big holiday the way she "always did," she would call her daughter, and her daughter had to take her to the market to buy food for the meal. The daughter was used to one-stop shopping: supermarket to the core.

Rebecca still shopped as she did half a century ago. She liked her individual butcher and bakery and fruit market. By the time her daughter had taken her from place to place she was so enraged she was barely speaking to her mother.

But the problem did not end there. Rebecca lives in a nice senior complex. When cooking time came the Chadult was brought in to help prepare the meal. She had to leave her spacious designer kitchen and work in a tiny kitchen designed for the efficient use of one or two elderly people—not for large-scale entertaining.

The two women would bang into one another and once again the daughter became enraged.

The final irony was that when the family came together, no matter how cold the air conditioning was or how many windows were open, the eating area and the living room were simply too hot and too small. The rooms would be packed to the rafters. People were irritable and couldn't wait to get out of there.

Although everyone would offer to help clean up, the kitchen area was much too tiny for that. So after everyone left, the daughter was once again pressed into service. And once again, she was enraged.

The question is obvious. How does the primary Chadult in an octogenarian's life allow his or her dignity to remain intact without being taken advantage of?

It is not an easy question to answer. But if no solution is found, the Chadult's anger will force the issue and all the parties involved end up the losers.

In this situation the daughter went to a support group and was offered some solid suggestions. She was drawn to one suggestion in particular. That was to begin slowly.

When the next holiday came around the daughter gave in on where the food was purchased. But then she stood firm about having the meal prepared at her own home.

At first Rebecca rebelled. That was to be expected. The daughter heard a lot of "but we always did it this way." The daughter stood her ground. She told her mother that times had changed and sometimes it is necessary to compromise.

While her mother pouted that whole first holiday, the change became easier with each subsequent gathering. This particular Chadult is a person who believes in peace at any price. But she reached the point where the price was out of range.

The issues are not limited to mothers. Fathers also need support.

Tom was faced with a parent problem, only from the male point of view. His father, James, had always been a proud man and always took pleasure in doing for himself. But like many men who are now in their eighties, he had never concerned himself with cooking and cleaning. That, after all, was woman's work.

When his wife died he insisted he could live alone and manage quite well.

Tom was concerned. When James retired years earlier, he and Tom's mother moved to a small town some fifty miles away. Now the old man was intent on staying in the home he had shared with his wife and not moving back to Tom's area.

Tom would call frequently. Sometimes his father was welcoming. Other times he would sound annoyed. "Why are you always checking up on me?" he would demand.

Although they had spoken frequently on the telephone several months passed before Tom and his wife, Angela, took a ride out to visit his father. James is a standoffish man and Tom is busy in a high-powered career. Time just drifted and the months elapsed as the Chadults went about their busy lives.

What they found distressed Tom and his wife. Nothing had been touched since his mother's death. Every room still contained her belongings. The house had not been cleaned. Cigarette ashes were everywhere, including some places where they might have proven hazardous. Dishes were piled in the kitchen and looked like they had been there for some time.

Tom, who had been raised to respect and fear his father, was simply struck dumb. He turned to Angela with a look of appeal. He hoped she would have a suggestion, because his father had always liked and respected her.

She nodded her head, understanding what was needed.

Tom's father had been standing at the door, arms crossed over his chest, with a furious look in his eye. "You're checking up on me again. I don't like it!"

His daughter-in-law smiled and took his arm. She led him into the kitchen and said, "I'll wash and you dry." The older man did as she said without uttering a word. She used the same technique—insisting that he help—as they cleaned the small house.

When they were through and Tom had carried out the last bale of trash, he told his father that from then on there would be help in the house weekly. Although James objected, Tom found a local woman through the church who not only cleaned but offered the old man some companionship. The arrangement worked so well that ultimately the two married—much to Tom's approval.

Dislike or fear of standing up to a tough father is not an uncommon experience. But at a certain time in life people find they have the ability to make necessary decisions. The condition of his father's house gave Tom the information that James needed help. He then used the best resource available to accomplish his goal. That resource happened to be his wife. Her way with James settled the older man down enough to allow Tom to tell him what needed to occur in order for the father to maintain his independence.

Tom also gained. He came away from the experience feeling less his father's son than his own person. It was a true win-win situation for all concerned.

Tom's father was unlike most older parents, who like the

idea of a daily call. What he saw as intrusion is taken by many parents as interest. How concern is shown or accepted is in the eyes of the beholder.

If your father or mother feels you are intruding in his or her life it is possible to say that you intend to continue calling and will only stop if he or she agrees to also call you.

A parent might want a daily call for the reassurance it offers. Recently there was a television commercial for an alarm device, in which an older woman screeched, "I've fallen and I can't get up!" That is a real fear. A valid fear.

Arthur, who is a widower, came home to the apartment in which he lived alone. As he closed his door he suddenly felt faint and fell to the floor. He stayed on that floor until the following day, when his daughter, Anita, who had a key, came by because he had not answered the telephone at their appointed contact time.

He was taken to the hospital and underwent many tests before doctors discovered he had suffered a minor stroke.

Probably this would rank high in any human being's list of fears. It certainly is way up there as we age.

Anita's experience in finding her father on the floor and knowing he had lain there all night is the kind of thing Chadults also fear. "Is my mother all right?" "I hope my father is managing."

We have been looking at Chadults dealing with parents who are single, whether through divorce or death or separation. Chadults are far more comfortable when both parents are alive and functioning as a unit.

When there are two parents the fear of something happening as it did to the man who suffered a stroke seems to have less urgency.

When there are two parents there is companionship. Even if they fought all through their marriage they chose to remain together. But this can bring up different kinds of problems. Chadults often feel it is their right to interfere in their parents' battles and relationship.

Carol and Dan constantly squabbled throughout their children's growing-up years. They would threaten to leave each other. Indeed, on several occasions Dan did walk out. But there was a bond that drew him back to his wife time and time again.

One day their Chadult son walked in when they were hurling dreadful insults at each other. They were saying absolutely hateful things, dredging up long-ago disagreements and angers.

The Chadult stood there for a moment and listened. Because he had seen so much conflict at home, he and his wife did not interact in the same manner. And from the lofty perch of Chadulthood he decided to teach his parents how to treat each other.

By the time he had gotten halfway through his "lecture," both parents were furious with him and told him to mind his own business.

He left in a huff and did not see his mother and father reach out to each other for hugs and closeness.

Again, the question poses itself. Would he have interfered in such a manner had the situation involved two friends, or would he simply have excused himself and come back at another, more convenient time?

There are other issues that will arise when a Chadult feels compelled to take action, and how the Chadult behaves the first time sets the tone.

One Chadult had to do some serious thinking about his role as a son. His father needed bypass surgery. Paul, the son, was not comfortable with the medical team his parents had always used. He had commented to them casually but repeatedly over the years that he thought it was time for a change. Neither parent wanted to listen; they liked their doctor.

Paul wondered if his parents just wanted to stick with the doctors they were familiar with. The parents were Polish and he was a first-generation American. He asked them if he could have another doctor come in just for a second opinion.

"That couldn't hurt," his mother said, and his father, already lying in the hospital, agreed.

Paul made some calls within his Polish community and found a doctor who was highly regarded and spoke fluent Polish—something the parents' longtime physician did not.

When the Polish-speaking doctor came to offer his opinion the parents were astonished. Here was a man who could speak to them. They didn't need to grope for words when they tried to explain symptoms and fears.

When the doctor was through with his examination he called the mother and Paul back into the room and told them their choice of surgeon was excellent. He asked them to call if they had other questions.

Paul was satisfied and the parents were delighted. Their permission had been asked. Real thought went into whom to seek out. The son's intervention was not done with presumption. It was done with respect.

But Chadults can sometimes act like children—not adult children but small children.

Four sisters, all married with growing families, decided their mother should no longer live alone. Sarah was a very special woman. She was clever and had raised devoted children.

Each daughter wanted Sarah to come live with her. It did not matter that one daughter would have to have three children share a bedroom, or that another was away at work most of the day, or a third lived on the fourth floor of a building with no elevator, or that the husband of the fourth strenuously objected to the proposed loss of his little television room. Each daughter wanted Sarah.

However, all Sarah really desired was a small place of her own. This was something that, with pooled resources, could have been possible. But the contest had gotten so intense that no sister was willing to back down. Finally, Sarah was forced to choose, and she opted to go to the fourth daughter's, where her son-in-law would not have his television room any longer. Her reason? It would afford her more privacy.

The upshot of this little story is that the four sisters did not speak to one another for years, until a family funeral brought them together!

Some people might call that mother love. Should we? If their mother was still capable of maintaining her independence, wouldn't allowing her that independence have been the greatest gift of all? Even if that independence was not financial, but Sarah could physically manage a small household by herself, would it not have been a great boost to her dignity?

Remember the son-in-law who was forced to give up his prized television room. How Chadults negotiate with their spouses when changes are beginning can determine whether we have a helpmate or yet another problem.

It is important to understand that when we are married there are certain decisions we cannot make alone, such as whom to invite to live with us or how we, as a couple, will spend our weekends.

Certainly it is important to spend time with our parents. But the decision about when to do so must include our spouse's input. When it does not we open the field for all kinds of anger. The battles may consist of silent brooding, rudeness to the parent, or deep resentment.

Barbara would always turn down invitations from her friends to go on long Sunday rides. She could never explain it, but a sense of nausea would overtake her. She never discussed this with anyone.

After yet another invitation drew the same response she decided to take some time to inventory her reaction. She recalled that her former husband used to demand that the family get in the car on Sundays and go for a ride; the ultimate destination was his father's house. The woman's father-in-law was a widower and these visits from his son meant a great deal.

But the drive was awful. The four children would be in the back seat quarreling and fussing: "She pushed me!" "She touched me!" "She's in my seat!" "I have to go to the bathroom!" When they finally arrived at her father-in-law's home Barbara was frazzled.

From her perspective, Barbara was ignored and her daughters were ignored. Her only function seemed to be to watch the children and prepare lunch for everyone—which she already did every day.

"What I wanted was for my ex-husband to be a father!" she explains. "He worked six days a week and rarely saw his girls. He was so focused on his visits with his father that he never seemed to give *them* the individual attention they had a right to expect.

"It was a frustrating time for me."

Her husband was an only child, and his ability to create a balanced life, one that more fully involved his four children, seemed impaired.

Indeed, being an only child in this difficult situation is fraught with distress. If an only child is fortunate, he or she has allies such as aunts and cousins to help share some responsibility.

But in the final analysis the parent wants the child to be

there. No matter that this child is fragmented and wants a life of his or her own. Being an "only" Chadult is a lonely job!

Evan has a father who is financially independent and well able to manage on his own. Even when his mother died, the Chadult did not overly involve himself in Ronald's comings and goings. He seemed fine.

The Chadult and his wife were caught up in work and family and social obligations. His wife, of course, had her own set of parents to think about.

One day Ronald, the independent father, had a stroke. It was not a major stroke, but the effects were permanent. He slurred his words, his hearing became impaired, and he was deeply frustrated and irritable.

He began to spend a lot of time at Evan's home. But after a while it became clear to Evan that this situation would not work. His own children were away at college or married, and he and his wife were enjoying that special time when they had more freedom to travel and visit with friends.

Ronald, despite his irritability, still wanted to be present when they entertained at home. He made it clear that he did not want to return to his own home with a nurse or aide.

The Chadult felt frenzied. His father was pressuring him. His wife was beginning to fret. He called his two cousins and asked if for a fee they would take his father into their homes.

"Absolutely not!" was the united response. "Why, he would make our lives as intolerable as he's made yours!" They told the Chadult, in effect, this was *his* problem. And indeed it was.

"You know, no matter which way I turned I was doing the wrong thing," Evan says. "I know that there are lots of battles between brothers and sisters, but the bottom line is I didn't even have the luxury of putting the issue in front of an equal. I had to do the deciding.

"What did I decide? Well, I decided he needed to go home. To his home. I got the best help available for him. My wife and I make it a point to visit separately and together so there are more visits. I did ask my cousins to stop over, and they have from time to time.

"What it really comes down to is I've got a no-win situation. I have just come to terms with that. I do the best I can. Sometimes less than the best, I guess. But I do go on from there."

There is a saying that a lot of parents pack up their troubles and send them off to summer camp.

But what happens when those "troubles" become adults and decide to move away?

Frequently, since our parents have given us both roots and wings, things fall into a somewhat comfortable pattern. For a number of years, visits back and forth become an easy routine.

But when we become caregiving Chadults, things change.

The comings and goings begin to diminish as our parents' capacity to earn funds or drive cars diminishes along with all the rest.

The end result is we see one another less frequently.

Sometimes there is great hurt. Indeed, the idea of "After all I did for my child during his growing years, look how I am being repaid" does cross many aging parents' minds. Sometimes it does not just cross, but remains there and festers.

Since most Chadults have some measure of intelligence— at the very least, we are able to take the emotional pulse of the people who raised us—we know we are causing disappointment. We know that day in and day out we are letting down the person or people who gave us life.

Especially if our mother or father is ill and we cannot be there as frequently as we would wish at such a time, we can be struck with intense guilt and sadness. What an uncomfortable and unenviable position in which to find oneself!

Choosing to move away is every adult child's right. But the time will come when we become Chadults and we must look at the consequences of our move. We may not like the way things have turned out, but we must remember that we have built our lives and must continue them.

Just as only children have particular problems to deal with, there are certain issues that arise when one child moves away while another remains at home.

There is a very delicate balance between siblings in this situation. The out-of-towner may be in a position to contribute financially while the local Chadult does the physical work. There are many cases where just this situation exists and seems amicable.

There are other situations, though, where gritted teeth are the order of the day.

Evelyn, who held down a full-time job, had an ill father. Not only did she have great stress at work, but getting proper help for Dad was an ongoing problem. People promised they would come for certain shifts, but then her father would call that the nurse's aide or home helper or other caregiver had not arrived.

Sometimes these calls came in the middle of the night. Others came during business meetings in the middle of the afternoon, and Evelyn would have to leave work because her father was incapacitated and could not be left alone.

Sheila, her sister, a wealthy woman, lived in another state. When she visited and saw the situation, she would subtly—so she thought—offer suggestions about making things easier. She would comment on the caregiver choices Evelyn had made. She would comment on the lack of cleanliness in her father's home.

As she did this, Evelyn, the in-town sister, sat and fumed, feeling worn and frazzled while her visiting sister carried an air of glamour and ease.

"Well, if you think everything is so bad, why don't you have him move near you?" Evelyn finally asked.

Her sibling raised an eyebrow in surprise. "What, and take him away from his home? That would be cruel!"

Evelyn turned on her heel and left the room, fearing she would say things she would later regret.

But she decided then and there she needed some help personally. She went to see a therapist who specialized in geriatric issues. She talked and cried and finally came to realize her father could no longer be kept at home under these conditions. She called Sheila and once again asked if she would consider having Father live near her. Once again she was told no.

"Making the decision was devastating," she says. "How could he have raised me and educated me and now when he needed me I could not give back to him? But I knew I was going to fall apart unless something was done, and finally I began making the rounds of the nursing homes.

"My sister was furious when I told her what I was doing. But with the help of my therapist I learned to respond to the guilt that I felt as well as the guilt being laid upon me."

In the end she placed her father in a nursing home that was close to her workplace. She had lunch with him daily. In the beginning he was withdrawn and angry. But nursing home social workers aided both her father and Evelyn during his transition.

The Chadult and her father now enjoy their time together more than they had in years.

Sheila, the out-of-town sister, still comes to visit, and she has learned to be more comfortable with the arrangement. She brings her father lovely presents and takes him out to dinner.

As time has gone on the two sisters have reconciled. Both now acknowledge the wisdom of the decision. The pressure is off both of them.

The true bonus is that their father is now being cared for consistently and he sees that his daughters are friends: "I was afraid of this nursing home business. I felt like I would be dumped here, but that's not what happened at all. My girls love me and Evelyn is less nervous. I'm still her father and I want what's best for her too."

Whether we face helping our parents with or without their consent, or have observed some of the early warning signs, or must make some tough decisions about their situations, there is a poetry and rhythm and grace within each of us. As Chadults we will find it helpful to discover that space within us that is given to kindness and love and beauty. The French writer Joseph Joubert, who died in 1824, could have been speaking for our age when he said: "You will not find poetry anywhere unless you bring some of it with you."

Many Chadults need to draw on this inner kindness when they "discover" that their parents are less than perfect, all-knowing beings.

When a son or a daughter becomes a Chadult the roles often reverse. The Chadult now has the power and sometimes Chadults are left wondering what to do with it.

Many adult children look at their parents and wonder why they were so frightened about a bad report card. Their parents now appear small and frail and simply unable to exert any control whatsoever.

Ideally, as Chadults we will view these changes with compassion and kindness and a touch of amusement. There will be little rancor, because hopefully, unlike the son who spent two hundred dollars a session to talk about his mother with a psychiatrist, we will have resolved any intense lingering angers.

There are many Chadults out there, however, who still carry with them the hurts and pains of their childhood. Most are married and have families of their own, yet they still have the excess baggage of that old business within their hearts and souls.

How then can they be expected to respond appropriately when they begin to see changes in their parent? How can they deal with the signs of deterioration and illness and fear of what the future holds, when the past still has a strong hold on them?

Most of us have seen examples of both types of Chadults. Certainly we are more comfortable around the former, even as we wonder at their capacity for forgiveness.

One woman was left at an orphanage when she was an infant. Although Louann was not mistreated, neither was she held and hugged and made to feel safe in the institutional environment.

She left the orphanage at the age of sixteen and, instead of finishing high school, found a job selling clothing in one of the better stores. She had one goal: she would make herself financially independent. To this end, she rented the cheapest room that was close to her job. She did not put in a telephone. Fortunately, her employers expected her to wear a smock, which they provided, so building a wardrobe was of no concern.

Louann was quite good at her job and quickly learned the styles and designers. She learned how to mix and match and create the most attractive look for women regardless of their height or size.

It was not long before she was a favorite among the ladies who shopped in the fine store.

One afternoon, after a long and tedious shopping experience, a woman named Mrs. Smith, who had taken a fancy to the young orphan, asked that Louann deliver the clothing she had ordered instead of shipping it to her.

She explained that she simply wanted to get to know Louann better.

Louann was flattered. Here was a woman she read about in all the society columns, and she was being invited to her home—even if it was only to deliver clothing. She could feel herself blush as she quickly agreed. She was given directions and wrote them carefully on her sales pad.

Suddenly she put her hand to her cheek. "Oh, my. I'm so sorry. I just can't do this."

"Well, why ever not?" asked the wealthy customer.

"I don't have a car. I know that's silly in this day and age. I don't even drive."

Mrs. Smith looked at the bright and sparkling young woman before her and sensed there was a story there. "Well, you said the clothes will be ready on Tuesday. My chauffeur will meet you at the front door when the store closes. How does that sound?"

"Heavenly," replied Louann, barely restraining herself from jumping up and down.

On Tuesday the clothes were ready and she looked them over carefully. She wanted to be certain everything was right.

She carried the heavy dresses to the front door of the store, and the chauffeur was indeed waiting for her in the sleek Cadillac limousine. He jumped out and took the dresses from her. She opened the passenger-side door in the front, but he shook his head. "I was told explicitly you were to sit in the back, and I always follow orders."

Louann watched the streets fly by; finally they arrived at the huge estate of her customer. They drove slowly and regally up the curved driveway. The chauffeur jumped out and opened the door for her. He then took the packages out of the vehicle. He pointed to the front door and told her to knock at it. "I have to use the servant's entrance," he explained.

Louann nodded and meekly made her way to the door. It opened almost immediately and a maid led her to a small sitting room, where Mrs. Smith waited with a china tea set in place.

"My son, Donald, is going to join us. I hope you don't mind."

"How could I possibly mind anything? I felt like Cinderella in your car. Thank you."

Just then the son came in the room. Louann was dumbfounded. He was the handsomest man she had ever seen.

Their eyes seemed to lock and the air seemed to stand still. Mrs. Smith watched the interplay and smiled with satisfaction. Her plan had succeeded. She had wanted these two to meet since she had known Louann. She had raised Donald with a strong sense of what a woman should be. She had been a working woman when she met his father, and she encouraged her son to look deeply into any woman with whom he became involved.

Time and again both his parents had reminded him that he did not have to limit his search for a bride to the narrow social set in which they traveled. Too many of the women seemed shallow and without purpose.

When Mrs. Smith first set eyes on Louann she had felt a pull. She had sensed this could be the woman for her son. She had gone slowly, however. She had wanted to be certain

Louann was genuine. She liked the younger woman's ambition and thoroughness. She liked the respect she showed all her customers. She especially liked Louann's quiet dignity.

She had no way of knowing that this dignity had been built as a defense against the emptiness and coldness of her childhood.

Shortly the three of them were talking over tea in a manner that would have surprised many who tried to climb the social ladder and become a friend of Mrs. Smith's.

Louann and Donald were soon very much in love. Not long afterward, they married, to the delight of his parents and the chagrin of the numerous society women who had hoped to make this incredible match themselves.

During their courtship Louann told Donald and his parents that she had been raised in an orphange. Without trying to elicit their sympathy, she expressed just what it had been like for her:

"They were never mean. It wasn't like Dickens or the movies. But they were indifferent. I never felt as if I had an anchor. Oh, it's hard to explain. But I do know one thing: I'm going to try and find my parents. I know they couldn't have done this out of cruelty. They must not have been able to care for me and did the best they could."

When Mr. Smith and his son looked at Mrs. Smith, they saw a rarity. There were tears on her cheeks. Mrs. Smith was actually crying. Now that was an unusual sight indeed!

"Mom, you sure brought home the goods, didn't you?" her son said as he took Louann in his arms.

Turning to his bride he smiled. "When I hold you like this does it feel like an anchor?"

Louann smiled. "Like an anchor made in heaven," she replied.

Soon after the wedding Louann began her search. She

was amazed to find that her new social standing opened every door. If her request was turned down by an agency or social service department she would simply tell her mother-in-law. When Mrs. Smith Senior got on the phone there was no nonsense.

In short order Louann found her mother. She still lived in the same city, but in the poorest part of town. She was a seamstress who had never married Louann's father.

All the Smiths offered to accompany her when she went to see her mother, but Louann shook her head. "I need to do this alone."

When Louann reached the second floor of the walk-up, she recalled just for a moment how different her introduction to the Smiths' home had been. How different the entrance and the setting.

She knocked timidly and a small old woman answered the door. Louann saw that her hands were gnarled and that the small but clean apartment held a basket of clothing and a hanging rack. She wondered how those gnarled hands managed to sew.

"My name is Louann Smith. I'm your daughter."

Cynthia stood stock-still in the doorway. She gazed in wonder at the beautifully dressed young woman who stood before her. "Well, it looks like I did you a favor after all," she said with no hint of welcome in her voice.

"But I'm your daughter. Don't you want to see me? To invite me in? Don't you have things to ask me?"

"Nothing that really matters to me. I dropped you off and that's that. I don't know why you came looking for me. I know you don't want money. What do you want?"

Louann turned her head away to hide her tears. This was hardly the way she'd expected the reunion to go. She had imagined being hugged and welcomed. Or, she had thought, possibly she would not be welcomed because there was another family and her existence was a deep dark secret. She had never expected to see a cold, indifferent, bitter person who did not care that Louann had found her.

Louann could feel her voice catch in her throat. "I don't *want* anything. I just wanted to find my mother. Why did you leave me in that place? Why didn't you keep me?"

By this time Louann had walked into the small living room and sat down on a rickety chair. She did not wait to be invited.

Her mother did not seem to care. "I didn't keep you because you were inconvenient. Single mothers didn't go on television talk shows in those days. How was I to go on? I could barely feed myself, let alone two of us. Your so-called father skipped out as soon as I told him I was pregnant. Besides, I'm not the kind of person who likes kids."

Louann did not even try to disguise her tears. She was simply inconvenient: that's why she had spent her childhood in a cold, uncaring institution. Inconvenient. She was beginning to shake, and she forced herself to take a deep breath.

"Well, you're *not* inconvenient. I'm going to move you to a nicer apartment and make sure you're taken care of. You don't have to like me. I wish you did. But you don't have to. Would you like to look for another apartment right now?"

Her mother was shocked. She had never received kindness in return for her abruptness. She had only known rudeness as a response to rudeness.

"Yes. I'll go with you," she said.

The two women were silent as they went to three different places in a much better neighborhood. They selected the nicest one. Louann told her mother she would furnish it and make sure her needs were met. "I don't think you should be doing much sewing. Your hands look pretty arthritic to me."

"That'll be fine," said her mother

All the arrangements were made. Cynthia was moved into the nicer apartment. Food was delivered.

As Louann sat with her husband and his parents she told them the story—how coldly she had been received, how indifferent her mother had been.

"You know, dear, you can have a food service drop off things for her if it's going to hurt you like this," said the elder Mrs. Smith.

But Louann shook her head. "She may not like me. I may not matter to her at all. But she did give birth to me, and I guess I feel some sort of obligation. I guess I'll try to see her once or twice a week, if only for a little while."

She smiled then. "Don't even try to ask me why I feel compelled to do this. I just do. Donald, you don't mind, do you? I—I just need to."

He gave her another of his big bear hugs. "I don't mind at all. You wouldn't be my Louann if you did anything less. Do what you have to do, honey."

Louann continued to make short visits to her mother. As Cynthia became more frail Louann hired aides to help her, and ultimately when her mother needed nursing home care she made certain the home was a good one. She continued visiting her there.

Sadly, Louann never got anything positive back from her mother. The old woman never melted even a little. The person Louann first met was the person who remained. But when her mother died Louann could feel warm about herself. *She* had done what was right. How it was received was not her issue. She had been blessed despite her mother's actions. The Smiths loved her and gave her the sense of well-being she had so long been denied. The more they saw of how she dealt with her mother, the more they loved her and wanted her to be happy and secure. So perhaps, without wanting to, her mother had served a fine purpose after all.

There are other responses, of course, to such situations. Seeing a person who is helpless can bring out the bully in some people.

Unfortunately, any number of frail old people are living in their children's homes at the mercy of Chadults who only care about Social Security—their parents'. There are endless ugly stories about malnourished old people who lie on soiled sheets in back bedrooms, their sole purpose seemingly to sign over the Social Security check when it arrives.

Perhaps some of these people were not kind and loving parents when their children were growing up. Perhaps they were abusive, and their Chadults now feel justified in turning the tables. But is there ever an excuse for cruelty? This is an argument that may never have an end. But old, defenseless people are just as victimized as abused children. Their plight seldom sees the light of day. Rarely are their stories newsworthy—especially if there is only one person involved.

Bob who worked for the power company was called to a home because the owner smelled gas. When he got there the owner's young son let him in, as his father was not at home.

The power company employee took his meter and began checking all the rooms in the house. As he started toward the back bedrooms the boy started following him. "It's okay if you go into these two rooms but you're not allowed into that room," he said nervously.

Bob looked at the boy and smiled. "Don't worry, I won't touch a thing. I do have to check each room. You can never tell with gas, you know."

"Well, my dad said not to let you go in there."

"I guess he'll just have to complain to my office. I need to check the entire house."

The other bedrooms were checked and then the power company man turned the handle on the door of the forbidden bedroom. He said later that his first reaction was olfactory. The smell was beyond anything he had ever experienced. He had been in many homes, but he had never smelled anything so vile.

There was a tiny light in the room and the shades were pulled shut and nailed to the windowsills. He would have walked away after checking the gas meter, but he heard a slight moan.

He turned to say something to the boy, but the boy had suddenly run away crying. The man ventured further into the room and to his horror saw a tiny, thin woman lying in the bed. She was surrounded by soiled sheets that had obviously been that way for some time.

Bob walked over to her and she reached out a frail hand, whimpering. He knelt by the side of the bed. "Don't worry, I'll get you some help."

He left the apartment immediately and called the police from the nearest telephone booth. He sat in his vehicle until they arrived, followed by an ambulance.

Not long afterward he saw the tiny woman carried out on a stretcher.

The woman was placed in a nursing home by the social service agency of the city, and after some time elapsed she shared her story with the nursing home social worker. It seems her son wanted nothing to do with her except her Social Security check. She was a virtual prisoner in the home, which she owned. Occasionally her grandson would slip in and give her some extra food, but most of the time she was kept alone in that dark fetid room—until the man from the power company came to check the house.

This is not an isolated situation. There are endless stories like it. Frequently these old people end up in nursing homes. If they are fortunate the homes offer counseling as well as food and shelter.

While we cannot assume that a woman of advanced years will have the time to work through and learn forgiveness, she may still ask the social worker to call her son and have him come to visit.

Sometimes the level of a parent's love and capacity to forgive can be boundless. Forgiveness brings its own magical power. It *may* heal the breach but it *certainly* will heal the person who has learned to let go of anger and betrayal and disappointment.

We have seen the examples of two extremes of behavior: a daughter who was willing to forgive her mother for abandoning her, even though the mother continued to show indifference, and a bullying son who kept his mother a prisoner, while the mother still wanted to see him.

Mental health people seem to have few answers as to why children interact with their parents as they do in such extreme situations. As one psychologist puts it, "You just have to know that each situation is separate and has to be handled one problem at a time."

Both the daughter and the son were in places of power. How each chose to use that power was obviously very different. It has nothing to do with gender. It is not necessarily the case that all females are natural nurturers and males are harder and tougher.

While the son ended up facing criminal charges, most Chadults never reach such dreadful extremes.

There is a story about a shoemaker who was working by the light of the stump of a candle that would soon burn out.

One of his coworkers commented, "It's a pity you won't have time to complete the repair."

"Don't worry," replied the shoemaker, "as long as the candle burns there is still time for repairs."

One of the people standing in the shop happened to be a priest. He was taken by the shoemaker's response and on the following Sunday he made it the thrust of his sermon. He said, "As long as the candle of the soul burns there is still time to mend our ways."

The same applies to dealing with our aging parents. As long as they are still alive we, as Chadults, have the gift of time. We can still make changes—treat our parents differently, be more attentive.

There is still time to mend our ways when we feel guilty and resentful because our parents are disappointed that we do not spend more time with them. We can have honest talks with them and come up with compromises. Remember, a compromise may leave everyone a *little* disappointed, but if we do not address these issues everyone is *very* irritated.

While our parents are still alive there is time to work with our feelings about having more power than they do. It is important that they not lose their status as parents. Since we walk more quickly and talk more quickly than they do, dealing with them can be like dealing with a child. Chadults must make allowances for the slowing down that comes with the aging process. If we continue to tie a child's shoes, the child will never learn to do it for himself. We must, as much as possible, give our parents the same freedom and dignity.

Chadults must talk appropriately about their parents' living arrangements. Whether Mom or Dad comes to live in the Chadult's home or other arrangements are made, these discussions can be held with kindness and caring. There need not be anger.

Independence is a precious thing to many people, regardless of their age. If circumstances show that Mom or Dad really wishes to live alone and is able to manage, there are all kinds of new devices to ensure they receive assistance if they are in trouble. There are buzzers and necklaces with buttons they need only push to summon help. If a parent values independence highly enough to risk living alone, it is worth letting him try to make his own life. But the Chadult needs to be part of that life by calling and visiting and showing concern.

Chadults, in this day and age, frequently have to deal with the issue of transiency. Sometimes it is the Chadult who has moved from the hometown. Sometimes the parent has retired to a warmer climate. With parent and child in different cities, good provisions can sometimes require creativity. But they *can* be achieved. Finding a guardian or a lawyer for the parent can often ease the difficulty should the parent require medical attention. There are times when quick decisions must be made and papers signed. Having someone close at hand to deal with such matters can be helpful in easing fears at both ends.

As in any human dealings, the best and kindest way is to begin slowly. Don't overpower your parent because you are used to having things done instantly. You may be able to call Japan and speak to a counterpart in business within moments, but parents require a somewhat different approach. They are older. They are generally set in their ways. You can't simply pick up the phone and "dial-a-solution." You may be surprised to find that when you go slowly, you can achieve much more.

Many Chadults say they felt clumsy at first in their caretaking. They had never before been in a position where *they* controlled their parent's destiny, and they felt the weight of this greatly. Many did not feel comfortable relinquishing their role as the "child."

There is something about taking over and guiding your

parent to decisions—or making those decisions yourself—that is unsettling. But as time goes on these situations do become a bit more comfortable.

There is a story about a man who worried about his deeds and would review his day at bedtime.

If he found he had done something wrong, he would say: "Jim, you're not going to do *that* again." But then he would catch himself and say, "Now, Jim, you said the same thing yesterday."

And he would reply, "Yesterday I wasn't telling the truth, but today I am."

In dealing with aging parents, as a Chadult puts himself through intense self-examination, he often finds that he did not live up to his own expectations. And, indeed, he can make himself promises that he does not live up to when the next occasion arises.

But to be human is to always strive to be better, to say that tomorrow I will make a greater effort to be understanding and attentive and concerned.

It is a great mistake simply to throw up your hands and think that there is no difference, that no matter what you promise, you will always fail. As long as you keep trying to do better and show good intentions, there is always room for improvement. You may yet get to that place inside yourself where you deal comfortably with a situation that is generally trying for most Chadults.

One of the difficulties of the time in which we live is the issue of how quickly things happen. We live in a time of instant gratification. There is instant oatmeal, instant coffee, instant communication, instant media.

When a Chadult deals with an elderly parent, learning to slow down is perhaps the greatest challenge. It may take Mom days to decide whether she wants to buy a dress, change apartments, come to dinner, visit a friend. Mom needs to have her own space and time to do these things. It is unwise to rush her. She might decide later that she did not think it through.

Now it's easy for us to think, "What is the big deal about whether she should have gone to visit a friend?" If you, the Chadult, lead a full and busy life, you probably would never give the question a second thought. But when Mom is old and has a great deal of time on her hands, she *does* give these things second thoughts. She will ruminate and brood, sometimes about things that to you seem small and insignificant.

That is why it is important, whenever possible, not to rush Mom. Let her go at a pace that is comfortable to her.

Because our lives are so hurried, it is possible that even in their old age our parents may still have a lesson to teach us. We can see them as models. They often can demonstrate that despite needing longer to get where they are going they still arrive at their destination.

Do *we,* as Chadults, need to keep our adrenaline pumping and rush our lives as we do? If we observe our parents and see that they still arrive at the destination even with their slower steps, can we, too, not learn the value of catching our breath and looking at what is around us? Could there not be value in taking life at a measured gait rather than always racing from place to place?

Chapter 2

KNOWING

THINGS WILL

CHANGE

---◆---

*Nothing in life is to be feared. It
is only to be understood.*

—Marie Curie

As our parents grow older we want to see them comfortable. When they are comfortable it offers us a sense of peace. We know they are housed and fed and secure in knowing we care about them. When our parents are comfortable we can more readily address the many issues that confront our own daily lives without having to worry about whether Mom and Dad's needs are being met.

Webster defines being comfortable as being in a state of ease.

Many Chadults may find it fairly manageable to ensure that their parents' existence is comfortable. But the question that presents itself is "How do parents feel about being in a state of ease?"

Pamela and Ben live on a manageable pension. Their home is paid for, their children are friendly and visit fairly often. To many of us this would sound like the ideal situation, the fulfillment of a dream we worked for all our younger years.

Their daughters, Laura and Linda, don't see this as their parents' dream situation, says Laura.

"They were active, vital people in the church community. They liked to camp. They enjoyed so many vigorous activities. Now, because they are so worried about their health, they do nothing but sit around. They have become so fearful that they worry about whether the food people bring to church suppers is fresh enough!"

Linda, her sister, echoes this complaint. "Their fear is so overriding that they are closing themselves off more and more. They even panicked when they heard my granddaughter had chicken pox. They were afraid I would carry it to them and they asked me not to visit until Robyn was better!"

Laura starts laughing. "You forgot it was even worse than that! Then they started worrying that you might come by just when Samantha caught it from her sister!"

The two women laugh. One points out that there are thousands of elderly people who are so anxious to have visitors, "and *our* parents bar the doors at the first sign of a germ!"

Certainly to some degree the parents' concerns cannot

and should not be overlooked. They are protective of their independence, and to them, illness equals loss of independence. In this they are not completely wrong.

But as in all things that are important in life, there must be balance before there can be comfort.

The parents have watched the changes around them, and for the most part they do not like what they see. Their friends are aging and dying. Many of their contemporaries who once camped and acted as Scout leaders are now bedridden.

While many parents perceive these events as very real "ghosts of Christmas future," their perspective is sometimes hard for the Chadult to understand.

When someone is forty or fifty and still working and vigorous, is it possible to relate to elders' fears, or even understand them despite having them explained?

Does someone twenty or thirty understand the concerns of the forty- or fifty-year-old who is worried about not having enough money to retire?

Many of us know the words and to some degree have an idea of what will transpire, but actually living the situation makes all the difference.

We have all heard people say, "I am getting old. I can't get around as well as I once did." We commiserate and sympathize, but until we are ourselves getting old we do not fully comprehend how it feels.

We have all heard Chadults talk about how difficult it is to find a good helper for Mother. We hear about Dad falling and needing surgery and a long period of rehabilitation. Again, we commiserate and sympathize. But until we are in the situation that requires us to change our life patterns to accommodate these circumstances, we do not know how difficult the sense of frustration and invasion and worry can be.

When we ourselves live through something, the immediacy of the situation is vastly different from when we are merely bystanders listening to a drama being played out.

Chadults must learn to make allowances and, yes, perhaps develop a sense of humor about these quirks in their aging parents.

We have all heard the saying "Judge not, that ye be not judged." But it may be equally important to remember what Cervantes said: "It is better that a judge should lean on the side of compassion than severity."

Most of us do tend to think others should do things the way *we* would do them, but we must never forget that it is inappropriate to judge. When we deal with our aging parents we should take a deep breath and accept them for who they are and what they have contributed to our lives.

There are, of course, some situations that are very difficult to accept. What if a Chadult was abandoned as a child, either figuratively or literally? What if a Chadult was abused as a youngster?

Does he or she owe anything to a cruel parent?

Much depends on how well the Chadult has come away from such a tragedy.

But very few members of the psychiatric community believe there can be true peace within ourselves until we have made peace with our parents. Sometimes the very thought of forgiving a cruel or absent mother or father is anathema to the victim. But if it is not done the victim continues to be just that—a victim.

It is not necessary to be friends when hurt has gone so deep. But it is necessary to forgive in order to make oneself whole. Anger can be a cancer that eats away at any joy we might experience. And it is possible that there is no greater anger than that of a wounded child.

"Revenge is sweeter than life itself. So think fools," said Bertrand de Jouvenal.

Forgiveness may be one of the hardest tasks any of us can pose for ourselves. How do we learn to forgive our parents for the taunts and real or imagined affronts that ultimately worked their way into the kind of people we became?

When we learn to forgive and truly feel the power of forgiveness, we know that now at long last we are in control, and the feeling of victimization may slowly lessen. Forgiveness cleans out the cobwebs. To forgive generally means to pardon or overlook an offense and to treat the offender as not guilty. When we can do that, we can make rational decisions about whether we wish to be involved with our parents.

Sometimes forgiveness can be helped along by allowing balance to enter into our judgment. It is helpful to weigh the good against the bad. What our parents did right is certainly as important as what we believe they did wrong. In 1849 John Greenleaf Whittier wrote an insightful poem entitled "Forgiveness," which explores just how important the need for balance can be.

> *My heart was heavy, for its trust had been*
> *Abused, its kindness answered with foul wrong;*
> *So, turning gloomily from my fellow men,*
> *One summer Sabbath day I strolled among*
> *The green mounds of the village burial place;*
> *Where, pondering how all human love and hate*
> *Find one sad level; and how, soon or late,*
> *Wronged and wrongdoer, each with meekened face,*
> *And cold hands folded over a still heart,*
> *Pass the green threshold of our common grave,*
> *Whither all footsteps tend, whence none depart,*
> *Awed for myself, and pitying my race,*

Our common sorrow, like a mighty wave,
Swept all my pride away, and trembling I forgave!

Whittier's overview of life could well serve as a lesson and reminder about what is really important to all of us.

Few people live in an intimate relationship, such as parent and child, sibling and sibling or, for that matter, husband and wife, without at some point feeling anger about something. Some issue is bound to arise that will bring strong emotions. Sometimes we are able to resolve those emotions in short order. By talking or perhaps writing about them we seek resolution. Fortunate are those who find it!

All too often, however, we do not handle things immediately or appropriately. We hope that the issue will resolve itself. As most of us know, the noise may die down, but the issue lies dormant, waiting to rear its head once again at a vulnerable time. If it is still lying there, we have not forgiven.

It is hard to imagine anyone being the kindest and best caregiver if that person still carries animosity in her heart. If she can remember more that was wrong than right, she has not forgiven. When the time comes that she is called upon to help her parent, she will be vulnerable.

Forgiveness is truly the cornerstone of being a good caregiver. Because only when we have forgiven can we offer care without resentment and the sense of being imposed upon.

Perhaps the time of greatest vulnerability is the time of change, the time when Mom or Dad must relinquish the role as parent and become the dependent of the adult child.

The parent is vulnerable as he or she begins to understand the magnitude of aging and its accompanying losses.

The Chadult, too, is vulnerable when he or she witnesses the changes in a once self-actuated person who is no longer able to function as in the past. Even though in many cases these changes are small at first, adult sons and daughters cannot help but be made aware when the changes affect them.

Dorothy, who has always prided herself on her housekeeping and chided her children when they were young about remembering to remove their shoes, had areas on her oven door that were marred by fingerprints. This would have been unheard-of even five years earlier.

Connie, her daughter, noticed the marks and quietly removed them when her mother was out of the room. She decided not to call attention to them even though she could have joked with her mother about "slacking off on the job." She feared Dorothy would be distressed or even angry—both at the marks, and at her daughter for noticing and then mentioning them.

These times when things begin to change are indeed tricky. Parents feel threatened. Their world as they knew it seems to be disintegrating. Things they took for granted, such as going for a brisk walk, quickly changing bed linens, repairing a hanging gutter on the outside of the house, climbing a ladder to repair a fixture, are no longer "no-brainers."

The walk will be less brisk. It will become more of a stroll. Changing bed linens may become a two-person task because lifting the mattress even slightly is more difficult.

When eyesight becomes poor it is harder to place a nail exactly where it belongs, just as it is more difficult to climb a ladder to make that repair or change a bulb in a fixture twelve feet off the ground.

One of the most common expressions people hear and repeat to one another is "Well, they did the best they could." If it is said to an unreceptive person the effect is like that of a red flag on a bull. Not only do we close down but we become inflamed. For many of us "the best they could" is simply not good enough.

However, as time goes by and we go through life and make our own mistakes and have our own regrets about what we could have done differently, we learn that people doing the best they can is what life is really about. Learning to forgive others and ourselves can be the greatest change we ever make. When we can do that there is nothing we cannot conquer.

Children who have been cruelly victimized by parents can find much to help their healing in therapy and in support groups. There is also an exercise that can be done in the privacy of the Chadult's home. Remember, the purpose of doing this is not only to aid the *parent* but also to make *oneself* whole.

Pick a quiet time without television. Take a sheet of paper and write a Forgiveness List. Take your time, because your thoroughness is important. The things you mention may be minor. "I forgive myself for not putting my shoes in the closet." They may be major. "I forgive myself for taking the car without permission." Write out your offenses—as many as you can remember. This will help cleanse your soul.

Then write a list of things you believe have been offenses against you. Offenses against you may also have the same range. "My mother made me wear boots and I was embarrassed at the party." "My father beat me with a strap and didn't even believe I hadn't taken the money."

Once you are done with your thinking and writing—this will not be a onetime process—begin another list. This is your Thankful List. Be just as complete. Like those on the Forgiveness List, these items may range from small to large, from trivial to life-altering. List all the things for which you feel gratitude.

Once you have looked at the Forgiveness List long enough, you may even choose to burn it. Or you may wish to keep the list to do a periodical personal inventory of your development.

The main goal here is to learn to focus on the Thankful List. As time goes on you will learn there is much in life to cherish and be thankful for, and your list may grow.

The author of Ecclesiastes wrote, "To every thing there is a season, and a time to every purpose under the heaven."

One of the many issues Chadults face is the question of timing. It is not only a matter of whether to intervene but of *when* to intervene.

In order to allow our parents their full measure of dignity, is it appropriate to wait until the need is dire? Do we step in sooner and begin making decisions for them that will alter their lives, even before they may be ready for such intervention?

Many Chadults have been caught in this bind. Mary said she literally used to grit her teeth to keep herself from picking up the litter in her mother's home when she came to visit. She had tried it once and her mother had become furious.

"Listen, young woman, I cleaned up after you all your life," she huffed. "I am the mother here! If you want to visit, that's fine. But leave my house alone!"

The onslaught was so sudden and fierce that Mary stammered an apology. "I only wanted to help."

"You can help me best by letting me do for myself."

On the other hand, John who was visiting his father watched as the older man raked the leaves in front of his house. This task had always been a source of pleasurable relaxation to the father, so John thought nothing of sitting on the front steps and visiting as the older man worked.

"You turned out to be one lousy son, I'll tell you that," said the father, his face red with fury. "After all the things I did for you as a kid, how can you sit there and watch me work this hard?"

This situation is something like the story of the woman who was describing the marriages of her two children.

"My daughter is married to a saint." She sighed happily. "She has full-time help. He insists he wants her to relax and enjoy her life. He pushes her to buy clothes all the time. He hired a laundress so she doesn't have to iron. Every night he comes home and makes her a drink and takes her out to dinner."

"He sounds wonderful," her friend exclaimed.

"Well, he is. But my life is not totally filled with joy. Take that woman my son married. She doesn't lift a finger in the house. She brought in a full-time maid to pick up after her. Like a little housework would kill her! She spends every day shopping and spending and spending my son's hard-earned money. She doesn't even pick up an iron to press a shirt. Then, when my poor boy comes home after a long day at work, she sits there and lets *him—him,* mind you—make her a drink, and then she insists he take her out to dinner!"

Many things are about perception. The mother perceived her children in roles of entitlement. Her daughter was entitled to live in the lap of luxury. To have every need met. Yet, another female, her daughter-in-law, was seen as someone taking advantage of her son, who also was entitled.

Knowing when to step in can almost be an art. Delicacy is often required, particularly in situations involving alert aging people who don't want their independence tampered with until they are good and ready to have it tampered with.

According to many therapists and families, people generally find their way if the relationship has been a strong and intuitive one. After all, Chadults grew up in their parents' home. They spent their formative years there and tend to know what will be acceptable.

But there can come a time when despite the amount of

feistiness the parent shows the Chadult simply cannot leave them alone—whether because of her own needs or those of the parent.

If the Chadult is intervening to meet her own needs she must try seeking some help in order to balance what she is feeling with what is right for her parent. On the other hand, if she sees an absolute need to intervene because of a threat to health or physical safety, then her choices are more easily identified.

Helping Mother clean up some clutter may be a need of the daughter. But there is no question that if Mother leaves burners on and walks away she could be in a potentially hazardous situation.

Sometimes the wisest course is to sit down with a social worker or other mental health expert and air your concerns. An objective listener can ease a heavy burden and help you see the issues and choices more clearly.

Support groups for Chadults can be invaluable. It is in this context that concerns can be laid out. It is in this context that you are likely to hear your problem emanating from someone else's mouth. There is something wonderful about knowing you are not the only one agonizing over a situation. Very frequently solutions seem to fall into place as well.

Another advantage of therapy is that it gives us the chance to work through negative memories we may have about our upbringing. Our parents did too little. Our parents did too much. We were neglected. They hovered over us.

How do we react to all the years of our lives with our parents? Now is really the time to find out. Do "good" parents get rewarded? Do "bad" parents get their due? Again, we must not fall into the trap of making judgments. Remember, a parent can see herself as being one way while her son or daughter sees just the opposite.

But now it is our time. We are in the power seat. How will we handle all the old garbage that cluttered our upbringing and continues to clutter our relationship with our parents?

This, then, brings up the issue of letting go, which may be the hardest task of all. If we learn to let go of how often our parents disappointed or disapproved of us, or made bad decisions that hurt us or favored a sibling, our thinking process will be clear.

This is the step beyond forgiveness. The ultimate growth is knowing we have the power to let go of the hurts we feel. It may require therapy, group support, or the understanding of a good friend. Above all it requires a clear and determined willingness to make it happen.

When the bug comes creeping back into our heads, we must be able to call a halt and remember that *that* was yesterday and *this* is today. Today is where we have to live.

There is another benefit for the Chadult in letting go of old hurts. As we will see later, the more "garbage" we can release when our parents are still alive, the more easily we can mourn them when they die.

In effect, a Chadult who is working at letting go of old angers is putting some healing into the bank for use at a later time. Opening that bank account could be our wisest investment. It is very hard to yell and rant at a headstone. It is most helpful to make our peace while there is still time.

We may be angry, but it would be wise to do the little things that are expected, just as if we were in a loving relationship. Call and ask if Mom or Dad needs groceries. That task does not require deep dialogues. But it does give the Chadult something to hold on to later. Taking the parent to a doctor's appointment can also be helpful. It gives us the opportunity not only to do a task but also to get a better handle on the parent's medical condition. There may be early warning signs of circumstances for which we should begin to prepare.

One of the most difficult problems Chadults face is the lack of preparedness for parental distress. Often we are so busy leading our lives and luxuriating in the pleasure of fewer demands that we do not take the time to stop and think, "What if Mother gets sick?" "What if Dad is incapacitated?"

Being prepared and reaching an understanding with an alert parent can serve as a buffer against future guilt and fear of making the wrong decisions.

One psychologist who works almost exclusively with the elderly says it boggles her mind that she is most often called in *after* a crisis has occurred.

"We are talking about intelligent people," she points out. "People who planned their pensions and their lives. People who raised children. Who nursed them through illnesses. Now, when it comes to the time of life where *they* have to be cared for—well, nothing was ever discussed."

This psychologist says that frequently people plan for how to dispose of their life insurance, their stock portfolios—all of their property. But the one matter we fail to discuss freely is our wishes in the event of illness.

"For goodness' sake," she urges, "get your adult children off the hook and tell them what you want!"

She makes a very good point.

Many of us enter into dealing with other people's business very timidly. How much more is this the case when that other person is our parent? We maintain, in our minds, the roles we and our parents have always played.

When we say "Mom" or "Dad" we don't picture a little child in a sandbox. We almost always envision the person who raised us. Who taught us right from wrong. The person who was taller than we.

Many Chadults say openly how out of character they felt when they began calling the shots. "Mother, what should I wear to school today?" became "Mother, it's cold outside. You'll need a coat!"

The role reversal can be shocking. And the new role is one none of us is really prepared for. We all know, at some level, that our parents are aging. We know this because *we* are aging. Our children are aging. Nevertheless we carry a longing for permanency that stops many of us from realizing that our parents are indeed growing old.

How can we help ourselves as we watch the process? How can we help them?

One social worker says the most important gift we can give our entire family is the honesty of recognizing the reality of the life cycle.

Many Chadults have double emotions when we begin to see the signs of aging. First we realize that our parents won't be around forever. Then the second realization begins to take form: Neither will we. If we really allow ourselves to observe them and see the way our lives will parallel theirs, then it is possible we might panic: "Is this how it will be for me? Am I really going to get old, too, one day?"

It seems completely obvious that this will be the case. But knowing the obvious and actually living it are not one and the same. We think *our* situation will be different. When we marry we generally say "for better or for worse," but we picture "better."

Probably all young brides and grooms imagine that the sweetness of the wedding day will carry on for the rest of their lives.

Those of us who have lived a few years more know this is far from how things really turn out. We know we have petulant days. Angry arguments. Hurt feelings. Business disappointments. Unmet expectations. Relationship disappointments.

Most of these things are part of the life process.

As children we watched our parents grow through all these events. We probably saw a mixed bag of reactions. We saw dignity. We saw anger. We saw hatred. We saw divorce. We saw forgiveness. We saw kindness.

We saw the entire spectrum of the human condition within the four walls we called home.

Perhaps the most painful thing we saw was our parents being angry with each other. This might have been more painful than when they were angry at us.

Did we run to our rooms and hide? Did we leave the house? Did we cry? Did we discuss it with our siblings?

We all probably did some of each. But the thing we did least was get involved. Most Chadults who are willing to recall such memories know this is the part of life that was most fearful. After all, this was parents' work and parents' business.

Now that we are grown we see things differently. We see more from the vantage point of being adults. Of having been through some of the experiences ourselves.

One psychologist observes that it is not uncommon for older couples to become irritable with each other, but he doubts such irritability begins in later years. He says the feeling has probably always been there, but it was masked because the couple was busy with their lives.

Things appear to unmask themselves as we age. Did we always have wrinkle lines just waiting to make their appearance?

Many Chadults have been faced with walking into their

parents' home and sensing a particularly disturbing sourness in their behavior. Dad crabs at Mom, and Mom at Dad, and we feel helpless watching. This behavior is not new—we probably grew up with it—but now that we have our own lives we see it in a different light.

Don't most of us, after all, go into our marriages vowing not to repeat the mistakes of our parents?

It is possible we have grown away from what we saw at home but the familiarity of what we saw does not leave.

We can either think to ourselves, "They're at it again," or we can leave the house feeling helpless. We erroneously believe those are the only two choices. A third might be to invite one of the parents out of the house for an hour or two. Run some errands together. Break the tension without ever referring to it. That is always an option.

Steven walked into his parents' apartment and said he could cut the atmosphere with a knife. There was no yelling. No one was saying anything mean, but the tension was there.

It brought back to Steven childhood memories of walking through the door and feeling the same way. He looked from one parent to the other and shrugged his shoulders. "Nothing's changed, I see."

"What do you mean by that?" his father snapped.

"Oh, this is what it was always like. You two on edge. Getting ready to fight or argue. Sometimes it's hard to think of visiting the two of you when I know this is what I will find."

There was dead silence. This was their only child, the father of their beloved grandchildren. And he said it was hard to visit their home?

"But, son, what could you possibly mean?" asked the father.

"Just what I said. It's hard to come here knowing how you two always act toward each other."

Although his parents were old and fairly set in their ways, both of them knew truth when they heard it. They began asking him some questions about what he meant. For once, instead of leaving, he expressed his feelings. When he was done they appeared to understand that he didn't come to visit out of love but merely out of duty.

Steven and Melanie, their daughter-in-law, shared the outcome of that visit: "It was like a transformation took over. I don't know if they were afraid our visits would stop—and that would never have happened. But they seemed to take stock of their own desirability. The next time we visited they were smiling and more outgoing than we could remember."

That does not mean that parents must put up a façade. But sometimes if they stop and think about how they may appear to their children, they can certainly create a better environment for those precious visits.

To recall the image of the bank account we are building for later in our lives—for that time when we are the aging parents—there are good investments we can make. We should remember the saying "Children learn what they live."

As they will someday be Chadults themselves, our children benefit from the examples we set with our own parents. Certainly no youngster comes into adulthood an exact replica of his or her parents. We are all variations on a theme. But some behaviors can be taught.

High on that list is responsibility. If a grandchild has been away at college for six months and comes home for the weekend, we can only hope that we have set the tone for him or her to visit Grandma. How nice if he or she does it before we have to demand it!

To instill this sort of behavior and attitude in our children, we have to begin early. Certainly older children can learn to visit. But how much more wonderful if the urge has long been there. The willingness. The lovingness.

It must be remembered that visiting does not have to be seen as a chore. It can be great fun, if Grandma is well.

There is a story about the great Supreme Court justice Oliver Wendell Holmes. He and another judge used to take walks every afternoon. One spring afternoon the two men were out walking when a beautiful young woman crossed the street in front of them. Justice Holmes, who was then ninety-two, stopped short and gazed after her in frank admiration.

Then he turned to his friend and said, "Oh, what I wouldn't give to be seventy again!"

To some of us seventy might seem old. But as medication and better nutrition become more and more a part of our lives we can hope that many of our parents will long continue to be active and spry and full of as much vinegar as Justice Holmes.

There can be laughter and fun and movies and restaurants and, yes, even travel. Families who are able to enjoy these things for years and years are very fortunate.

But, as we know, that is not always the case.

For many people money is an issue. Not the unrealistic fear of poverty but the realistic fear of poverty. Most people cannot afford private nurses and aides.

Most Chadults were raised by parents who have an absolute dread and abhorrence of nursing homes. To the older generation this was the dropping-off place. It was the public symbol that no one cared. Frequently care was minimal and cruelty was to be expected.

Certainly horrid conditions still exist despite the best efforts of government regulators. But fortunately these are the exception.

Many of today's nursing homes provide full-time social workers and active family groups as well as support groups.

State and federal agencies make unannounced visits to homes to check on the level of care the residents now receive.

Those who live in nursing homes are no longer even called patients. They are "residents," because the nursing facility has become their home.

Resident councils have great clout in many homes. When the governmental agencies make their visits they listen with care to what they are told by the residents.

Another change in the entire nursing home picture is that more residents are alert. This can be a great bonus to those who would like both to live in memory lane and to stay current. Sharing memories of an era can be a satisfying pastime if listeners are receptive. Alert nursing home residents enjoy sharing experiences with others who were part of that time. While it is important to be aware of what is current, it can be comfortable to go back to the way things were.

Visiting hours are generally quite flexible and families are encouraged to attend functions established by activity directors.

While the private-pay nursing homes obviously have more amenities such as larger sleeping areas, more decorative settings, and perhaps more outings, money is not the sole factor in determining what a nursing home provides.

There is a saying among nursing home administrators that next to nuclear power no industry is more heavily regulated than the nursing home industry. This, in many cases, has proven to be a bonus. The unannounced regulatory agency visits, the guidelines for staffing, the quality of food, and the frequency of doctor visits all are under scrutiny.

Although a Chadult may still feel guilty if the funds are not available for private care, there is peace of mind in knowing that a mother or father can be cared for and made comfortable even when money is tight.

Should placing a parent in a nursing home become the course of action you must take, try to think ahead. We are all going to age. Many of us will become infirm. When Chadults see that happening to their parents, it is time to start research. *Don't wait until you are in the crisis. Bad decisions are made in such haste.*

Some Chadults see the signs and start looking around without telling their parents. In some cases this is wise. It is not always necessary to panic someone who is becoming more and more incapacitated.

When checking out nursing homes, make unannounced visits whenever possible. See how the home is really run. The disadvantage of this, however, is that you may find the admissions person too busy to sit down and answer your questions thoroughly.

You may walk into a home and smell strong odors. This does not always mean the home is badly maintained. Perhaps the smell from a very recent episode of incontinence has not yet dissipated.

On the other hand, sometimes odors can be a warning. This is one of those situations in which you must trust your sense of the people you meet. Make certain you meet the admissions director. If you spend time with the administrator, the director of the building, you will get a feel for how the building is run and how its occupants are perceived by the staff.

Also, make certain you meet the director of nursing, who is in charge of the residents' medical care. While a doctor, of course, does the prescribing, remember: this is a *nursing* home. The director of nursing should be knowledgeable and willing to listen and have a staff of nurses and aides who emulate her philosophy.

The hardest time to make a nursing home decision is

when Mother or Father has been in the hospital and you get a call from an overworked social worker saying your parent must be placed within a day or two.

If you find yourself in such a situation it might be wise to let yourself be guided by the hospital social worker. He or she will generally give you a manageable list of places that have space available and will have had experience in working with the nursing homes.

But as in any situation, time is the luxury. When you can take the time to do a thing well you will do it better! If you see signs that are troubling you, be certain you act on them now. Start visiting homes.

Marsha had two daughters. Her husband had left her when they were young. She picked up the pieces of her life and despite having no skill or experience went to work in a restaurant.

As the years went by she became its manager. Her children were able to make it through high school and get jobs of their own.

One day, this woman noticed that her hands had begun to tremble. She went to a doctor, who sent her for extensive testing; it was discovered she had Parkinson's disease.

She took the time to do her own investigating and made a decision on which nursing home she wanted. She simply would not allow her children to house her. They had their own families and she had grown much too independent.

Her children were pained as they watched her slowly deteriorate. They finally decided to speak with her about it.

"We could see it was harder and harder for her to manage and we felt we couldn't put off talking with her about it any longer," said one daughter.

"We went over there feeling like traitors," said the other. "She had done all she could for us, and here she was, alone.

Not living with us. Neither of us had a situation where that would have worked. My sister and I were in tears as we drove there. We didn't know what to say. We had no money to offer. Only our love.

"She saw our faces when we got to her apartment. She asked what was wrong. We both stammered and then tried to talk at the same time. We were trying to tell her we love her. We couldn't take care of her. We felt guilty. There were so many messages."

The mother responded with the same grace that had characterized her life. She saw their pain and smiled. "It's okay. It really is," she said. "I have already made my nursing home arrangements. I just want to be certain that you will visit me as often as you can. I had planned to tell you soon. But you stole my thunder."

The daughters were dumbfounded. They had any number of questions. How did you find the place? Why didn't you tell us? When can we see it?

The woman answered all their questions. The daughters' visit to the nursing home was not filled with the agony so many families endure. To the end this spectacular woman carried on her own life according to her own agenda, and she gave her children a great gift—freedom from guilt and the example of using personal power.

The daughters kept their promises to visit her frequently. Visiting is one of the few gifts Chadults without financial resources generally have it within their power to give.

Most often, even when the signs of lessened capacity for independence are there, decisions are put off because they are so painful. It is generally the Chadult who must raise the issue or break the news to the parent if the parent is still alert.

Perhaps in the final analysis, if the adult can do what this mother did by acknowledging and taking control of her situation and her daughters', it is the ultimate act of parenting.

Great philosophers throughout the ages have always noted that things change.

There is a Jewish tale about a rabbi who said he would never believe anyone who told him he was perfect: "If a king told me I wouldn't believe it. Even if God told me I wouldn't believe it. Because even if a person is without flaw he has no idea of how he will be a minute later."

It is no different with aging. You can feel hale and well, but a sudden slip on a patch of ice can change your life forever.

Chadults must understand the truth of this and live each day understanding the importance of letting Mom know they care. Letting Mom know there has been forgiveness. Letting Mom know there are some happy memories interwoven with the anger and disappointments they experienced.

When you know, really know, that things will change, it profoundly affects your actions.

Ken realized the truth of this when he was told his father had had an accident. The two had always had an abrasive relationship. And as Bill, the father, got on in years he would treat his son with insulting derision.

Then one wintry day Bill had an automobile accident. He was fairly badly bruised and was taken to the hospital. It was his first experience with ill health. All his life he had been strong and well, never even able to understand people who were laid up with the flu and missed work. "People like that are wimps," he would say.

When the police arrived at the accident scene they saw he needed medical attention. An ambulance was called and he was taken to the hospital. When asked who should be notified, he was startled. He had never been in such a situation. There had never been a need to notify anyone about him.

"Well, my son, I guess," he said and gave the police the information they needed.

When Ken was called he, too, was taken aback. His father needing him? He could not imagine sitting at the hospital bedside offering comforting words to the "old man."

But, like nearly every other Chadult when called, he went to the hospital.

He was shocked by what he saw. His father had sustained some head injuries, although these had not affected his ability to communicate. Also, he had a broken leg.

"I still remember looking down at him in the emergency room," Ken says. "He looked a lot less cantankerous than I remembered him ever being. In fact, he looked almost glad to see me. Now, that was a new twist."

Ken says he was troubled by his own lack of feeling about seeing his father there. Their relationship had been bad for years, practically all his life, and he saw his father as a near-stranger who was not well.

But sometimes good can come from the most unlikely incidents. Bill's hospital stay was long. Day after day he lay in his bed, without visitors except for the nurses who came to give him shots and pills and check his vital signs.

He had a long time to reflect on how he had conducted his relationship with his only child, who stopped by just briefly once or twice a week. He saw that as the father he had established this underlying warfare in motion. He had been the pace setter and what he had set in motion was now there to haunt him.

Ken, too, had a lot of time to think. Although he did not visit as attentively as some sons might have, his father was certainly in his thoughts. He saw how differently his friends treated their mothers and fathers. He saw the level of concern they felt. He did not like this void in himself, this sense of seeing his father not as a parent but as a stranger to whom he paid only a modicum of attention.

These thoughts would come unbidden to his head as he drove around on his sales calls. Finally, he decided to do something about the situation.

He had no idea if his father would be receptive, but he knew *he* had to try.

When he got to the hospital that evening there was no one else in his father's room. He looked at the man, still bandaged, leg in a cast, and decided he would cross the line and try to fill that void with caring.

His voice was gentler, his demeanor softer, as he sat down on the uncomfortable visitor's chair. "So, how are you, Dad? Any better?"

Startled, Bill looked at him. Ken had not used such a warm tone of voice since this whole ordeal had begun.

But Bill was wise. Rather than making some snappy answer such as "Why the sudden change?" he took the kind question in stride.

"Some days are better than others, I guess." His tone was not edgy. He was not waiting for the next barb to fall. Ken noted the difference in the response. He had heard only sharp, angry, sarcastic responses all his life. Here, finally, he was getting an adult to reply like an adult.

Ken did not stay long that evening. But when he left he leaned over the bed and touched his father's shoulder in a caring way. With some difficulty his father reached over and patted his son's hand.

They spoke no more, but each felt a slight whisper of change had occurred.

Ken drove home feeling somehow pleased. He had no illusions that a strong and intense relationship could be built, but he felt after the visit that perhaps some of the angry edge would be softened in his interactions with his father. He felt good about initiating the change, and he also felt good about his father's response. A turnabout in their relationship had begun.

Anyone, Chadult or otherwise, can only benefit when he understands that not bringing goodwill and positive feelings into important relationships means that he is cheating himself.

There is an old saying: "One is not permitted to cheat another. Even more, one may not cheat oneself."

When all of us acknowledge that parents will age, possibly be infirm, and will die, we may attempt more vigorously to keep our relationships healthy. When we are surrounded by good feeling toward and from the people we love we are in little danger of cheating ourselves.

But all this is in the knowing. The knowing with certainty that we *will* see changes. Not "we might." We *will!*

It would be wise to remember this when dealing with siblings and in-laws and spouses. If you are the one to have come to understand this first, then it is important that discussions begin with these family members *before* they become urgent.

Newly married couples who talk about having children and building careers and buying homes would also find it useful to talk about what happens when Mom or Dad is old or widowed. "As my mate, what part do you think you can play as my support or hands-on helper?"

Since the issue of aging parents is almost inevitable in most families, why is this discussion not held in the early stages of a couple's relationship? If we prepare ourselves early and look at the long view, then when the time comes there are fewer surprises.

All too often the question of what to do about Mom comes to the fore only when Mom is in crisis. In such a situation, there is no orderly transition and the spouse is often not involved in the decision-making. This inevitably leads to resentment and can make any sane person feel torn apart.

One couple, Len and Nancy, was faced with trouble when Len's mother had a stroke and could not be left alone. Her son had always promised she would never be placed in a nursing home, but he had never discussed this promise with his wife. They had never talked at all about the possibility of parental change and illness.

Unfortunately, money was very limited. There were not the funds for private help. The mother had to give up her apartment and come and live with Nancy and Len.

The daughter-in-law understood when she married Len that she was marrying an only child. But the ramifications of this had never really hit home.

The moment of truth came when Len told her of his promise and that he felt he had no choice.

At first his wife was furious. But then she saw he felt trapped into taking his mother to their home, and she, too, felt trapped.

Things became very harried when she realized he was going off to work as usual and she would be left at home to care for the older woman.

She became so enraged that she went to her parents' home for a week to sort things out. She cried and told her parents how unfairly she was being treated. She simply did not want to share her home or assume all the responsibility.

Her mother was a wise woman. She listened most of the week and let her daughter pour out her heart. But then after dinner one evening she asked her daughter a salient question: "What if it were me? Would Len take me in? Would you?"

Her daughter nodded. Of course she would take in her mother. "Well, why do you expect Len to love his mother less than you love yours? Why do you expect him to care less than you care?"

Her daughter had never thought of it that way, and they talked about what type of help she might seek from the community.

But there was a further benefit to the discussion. It gave mother and daughter a chance to talk about what they would do should either of the daughter's parents become incapacitated.

She called Len and asked him to come to her parents' house. There, the four of them talked about his mother and some alternatives—including day care and visiting hospital volunteers who could come and stay so the daughter would not be housebound.

They also talked some more about their own needs and wishes should such a situation arise in their lives. They hammered out an agreement, which they all hoped would never be invoked but which they understood they would honor should the need arise.

On the one hand Nancy got hit with a sudden, difficult situation, but on the other hand this situation forced her to think through in an orderly manner issues that she had never before faced.

When you know with certainty that things will change you have the "luxury" of being prepared and making the necessary arrangements.

This type of discussion should *begin* when children come of legal age. You, the Chadult, should take the lead. Both parents and children should acknowledge that in the inevitable course of life there will be a day when Mom or Dad is not a healthy, vigorous human being. This does not mean we need to terrify our young people or create great insecurities and apprehension in them. Rather, it means instilling a healthy and realistic preparedness. We are letting them know that things will change. We are telling them this change is normal. By beginning early, we may alleviate their fear of aging and what will happen when they reach that point of being Chadults with aging parents.

The other advantage of doing this is that children will hear it from you. If you explain the issues well, you may head off one of those difficult situations where siblings quarrel about who should be in charge of your care when the time comes.

These are issues that can divide families. In fact, that happens far too often. But if children begin to understand the concept of aging and change when they are younger, then they can grow up knowing each of them will be a part of your becoming old. They will know that all parts will not be the same, and by the time their help is needed, dealing with these issues will have become second nature to them.

One of the best ways to show your children how the generational process works is to let them see how you interact with your own parents, if possible. Let them see a level of interest. Let them see a reasonable pattern of visiting. Let them see and know when it is necessary for you to help your mother or father by driving them to a doctor or helping with the marketing. Let them see and hear discussions with your parents about their wishes. Do they hope to live independently? Is there the possibility or desire to live with you? How do they feel about nursing homes?

All these vital discussions can have the double benefit of preparing your children for the time—which will come— when they will be the Chadults and you the aging parent.

There is an old Russian tale about a husband and wife who sent their son to a bedroom to get a thick blanket.

"Why do we need this blanket?" he asked as he brought it to them.

"Well, it is that time when Grandpa is getting too old to take care of himself, or even to live with us."

The boy, who loved his grandfather, was bewildered. "Well, what do we need the blanket for?" he asked.

"Son, it is our custom that when someone gets old and unable to be a productive part of our society, we take him out onto an ice floe and cover him with a blanket so he will be warm until he dies."

The son was stunned. They were talking about his grandfather, who had taught him to play chess and talked with him—until just a few months ago, when the old man had regressed and become like a child.

"Well," he thought to himself, "if this is the custom, then it is what must be done."

With that thought in mind he went into the kitchen and brought out a pair of shears. Not saying a word, he took the thick blanket intended for his grandfather and cut it in half.

His father became quite angry. "Why did you do such a foolish thing?" he demanded.

"Well, Father, I was only following your example. I cut the blanket in half because it is a good, thick one. I wanted to save it for your turn!"

Perhaps all of us need to bear this in mind: children *do* learn what they live. Your actions can be their greatest teacher.

Just as "Be prepared" is the Boy Scout motto, so it could well serve most of us as a reminder when we are dealing with our aging parents. Being prepared goes hand in hand with knowing things will change.

Change need not be frightening. It simply is. If there were no change we would all still be in diapers. The seasons would not alter from the icy sculptures of snow-covered trees to the burning, passionate colors of autumn. There would be no high school graduations or beautiful weddings with brides going down aisles on the arms of their fathers.

Change is a necessary part of life and growth.

We cannot live our lives afraid that change will occur. When our children graduate from college and go forth into their chosen professions, we begin to see changes in how they behave.

Perhaps they exhibit a new assurance about the world that is most attractive.

When they marry and become parents, once again there is change. Once freewheeling young adults, they become responsible members of the community who attend PTA meetings, make certain their children are given religious training, and participate in extracurricular activities such as basketball and soccer and gymnastics. Our adult children worry about *their* youngster's reading and arithmetic and spelling. These children of ours, whom we couldn't get to sit still long enough to do homework, are now doing everything by the book.

They plan to raise perfect children.

And we are certain they will!

But we do watch all this activity with a raised eyebrow most of the time. For we have memories of our own.

Memories of trying to nail those now-diligent fathers and mothers down long enough to get them to do their homework or clean their rooms or do assigned chores.

But that is what change is all about.

One of the beautiful things about human beings is that they have the capacity to change once they have the will. They need not always be the wild rambunctious people they were when they were young. They can change.

Disheartened parents would do well to remember this. Far too many people see youngsters as somehow being locked in a time warp, forever unable to assume responsibility or take care of themselves.

Usually that is far from the truth.

People grow. People change. Life changes. Not all change is exciting and happy.

Sometimes, people grow and then they reach the point of aging. If they know it will happen to them—not just to the guy down the street—they can spend those growth years preparing for old age. They will be more comfortable and more at peace.

When we know things will change we can also learn to take joy in the moment. We can learn to appreciate what is good and happy in our world.

Knowing things will change can be exciting. There is a sense of adventure when we understand that there will be new challenges, that we will wake up each day not to the sameness of yesterday but to new experiences and new problem-solving opportunities.

When we know things will change we can look at those opportunities and build on them.

Most of all, when we know things will change, we can begin at any time—*now*—to make peace with our pasts and peace with our parents. If we can accomplish this we prove once again the benefit and importance of change. We need not be stuck in yesterday's anger and self-pity, even if they were justified.

When we know things will change, we know there is always hope. Hope that today and tomorrow will bring us kinder thoughts and greater wisdom and deeper caring, even if our parents were not all that they could have been. As Chadults, let's learn to be all that *we* can be!

Chapter 3

PERCEPTIONS

AND

OBLIGATIONS

◈

*Life is easier to take than you think; all
that is necessary is to accept the
impossible, do without the
indispensable, and bear the intolerable.*
—Kathleen Norris

While there are always new things under the sun, especially in the quickly changing times in which we live, there
are also some truths that have withstood the test of the ages.

The philosopher and mathematician Pythagoras lived in
the sixth century B.C. During the course of his life he traveled
extensively in the Middle East in quest of knowledge before
settling ultimately in the south of Italy.

According to Michel de Montaigne (1533–1592), Pythagoras once said, "Life resembles the Olympic Games. A few men strain their muscles to carry off a prize; others bring trinkets to sell to the crowd for a profit; and some are there who seek no further advantage than to look at the show and see how and why everything is done.

"They are spectators of other men's lives in order to better judge and manage their own."

Perhaps that is the real lesson for Chadults. If we are given the opportunity to witness the difficulties of others while knowing that they may be *our* personal experiences at some point, then observing and hearing what others have done can be of great value.

There is a saying that the family you come from is not as important as the family you are going to have.

Perhaps Bob serves as an example of just this fact. He and his father, Don, sixty-eight, had never had a strong relationship. His father had worked long and hard to provide for his family. But as in many homes of the older generation, they saw little of one another.

Bob, although told frequently enough that what his father was doing was for the benefit of the entire family, still felt the emptiness of not having both parents present at school functions and other events important to young people.

When Bob's mother died suddenly, the two men, nearly strangers, had to come face to face with each other in many ways.

Bob had been a Chadult for some time. He, unlike Don, was committed not to earning vast sums of money but to being a family man who was there for his children's ball games and recitals. He left, however, almost no time for his parents.

An only child, Bob now had to become involved with his

father. The first major project Bob could remember sharing with his father was planning the mother's funeral.

At that intense time of vulnerability, Bob noticed for the first time that his father was no longer the all-powerful man of means who had always been so strong and distant. Instead Bob saw him as a mortal who was now bereft. The concept of his father being bereft was startling to the son.

Bob was so shaken by this new perception that he did not know how to deal with Don. So he said nothing. After all, no easy lines of communication had ever been established. Certainly funeral planning does not lend itself to such an endeavor. So the two men made decisions, each keeping his emotions safely tucked away.

When they left the funeral home after making arrangements they shook hands, and each got into his own car. They planned to meet later that evening, when Bob would be bringing his wife, Sharon, and children to the visitation.

So accustomed was Bob to not being involved with his father that he never thought to invite him back to share the waiting hours with his family.

There were a great many people at the evening visitation. Many were Bob's and Sharon's friends. Many were Bob's children's friends. But there was also a strong contingent of people who came to see Don.

Somehow this surprised Bob. He had always pictured his father as a loner. Now here he was surrounded by a large party of people who seemed to know him well and have genuine concern for his well-being.

Bob still recalls looking at his wife and seeing his bewildered look mirrored on her face.

The evening went by fairly quickly. They were to meet again the following day. Once again the two men shook hands and went their separate ways.

The visitation next afternoon showed the truth of the saying about "the family you are going to have is more important." Things began to change. Bob's daughter, Jennifer, arrived from college. Nineteen and outgoing, she had never known her grandmother well. She was sad because she believed her lack of tears was a sign of disrespect.

Seeing that her parents were busy with some old friends, she walked over to her grandfather, who was sitting alone.

"When he looked up at me I saw my father's eyes on another face—a lost face," she recalls.

"Grandpa, I'm really sorry," she said. "You must feel so alone even though you have such a big group of friends. Mom and Dad said you had quite a crowd here last night."

"Please sit down for a few minutes," the older man said. "You're right, you know. I feel very alone. Those friends last night were mostly people from business. It's important to their careers to make this type of visit."

Jennifer detected the note of cynicism in his voice and felt uncomfortable. Nearly twenty years old and she couldn't find a common ground to speak to her own grandfather. Should she get up and leave him? No! That didn't feel right.

Instead she reached for Don's hand, and he willingly took hers.

They sat quietly for a while, and when some people came in to see Don she went to join her parents.

"That was very nice of you," her mother commented approvingly.

"I didn't do it for that reason. I don't really know why I went over, but he seemed so alone."

"My dad alone?" Bob said. "I've never even imagined such a thing. He was always so busy with other people."

At the end of the afternoon Jennifer told her parents she wanted to ask her grandfather to join them back at the house.

"Why, certainly he's welcome. But I don't imagine he'd be really interested," her father replied.

But Don *was* interested. Jennifer drove separately with him and they spoke very little. Again she felt uncertain about how to break the ice.

When they got to the house there were no visitors. Jennifer and her brother, Kenneth, a high school student, sat with their parents and grandfather.

"This is the part that chokes me up," says Bob. "Here my daughter easily glided through a barrier that looked like sheet metal to me all my life."

Once back in her own home, where she felt more at ease, Jennifer spoke naturally with Don. She asked him about his life with her grandmother. She pulled no punches, although she was kind. "You know, I really know very little about you. We never had a real sense of grandparents from you two. Now I'd like to know you better so I don't lose more time."

To Bob's astonishment Don began to cry. He didn't utter deep, racking sobs, but tears streamed down his cheeks.

"In all my life I never wanted this to happen," he said. "I have one son. I did what my father did. Made sure he had everything he wanted or needed. That's what fathers do!"

Sensing the tension rising in her husband, Sharon laid her hand on his arm.

"Well, fathers do lots of things," Jennifer said calmly. "You know, Grandpa, this could be a new time for us. We still have time to get to know one another—and if I do say so myself, we're a pretty terrific family!"

Don looked at his son tentatively. He detected nothing from him that added to this opening.

"Son," he said, looking his only child in the eye. "Would I be welcome to visit here?"

"You know, Dad, it's been so many years. I just don't

know what I feel about this new family spirit thing. I guess I got too old begging for your attention."

Once again the tears streamed down Don's face. "I guess you did. Sometimes people make choices and they are not always the best ones. I will be sorry for this all the days I have left."

"Hey, now, just a minute," Jennifer put in, perturbed at her father's reaction. "I'm part of this family too. I want to see my grandfather. If I can't do it here I'll just visit you at your home. I want to know you."

"I would like that too," said Don, this time taking *her* hand.

Bob sat there with all the years of his life flashing before him. All the missed events that should have been shared. All the feelings of rejection. All the pain. Even now that he was a man in his late forties, it hurt him just to remember.

But then he looked at his glowing daughter, and he felt a certain pride in what she had become. Perhaps a different father would not have produced a son so dedicated to his family. Perhaps Jennifer would have been different.

In any event, the decision was taken out of his hands when Jennifer said, "Let's have lunch next Monday. I'm out of school on break."

Kenneth, more introverted than his sister, had been silent, but now he suddenly spoke up. "I'd like to come too, Grandpa. It seems like we have a lot of catching up to do."

Bob did not offer to join them. But he knew the children were in contact with his father, and after a time he began asking about him.

After a year Don became seriously ill. He needed bypass surgery. That was when Bob decided to take matters into his own hands. He called his father and arranged a dinner just for the two of them.

They avoided emotional issues at first. But finally Bob, using a gentle voice, told his father he had been working all this past year on putting behind what was past. "I don't know if I can ever really let go of all of it, Dad, but I feel we have some starting place now that good old Jenny got involved."

The older man smiled. "She's quite a gal. She thinks the sun rises and sets on you, you know."

"Yes, Dad. I *do* know. I'm lucky about that."

"No, son, there's no luck involved. We all make choices. I just wish mine had been wiser. No matter what I have accrued you have infinitely more."

That was the only conversation the two ever had on the strained relationship. It would have been unrealistic to think that a lifetime's worth of barriers could all be knocked down in a day or a year. But at least the two men could visit. The entire family was there when Don had his surgery, and they visited regularly during the recovery period.

While Bob and Don would never have deep father-son intimacy, thanks to the efforts of a third party, which led to their own developing relationship, they now had a sense of family.

As time went on the children convinced Bob to include his father in holiday celebrations. At first Bob resented this greatly. His children were now both away at school and he did not want this "intruder" sharing precious mealtimes that had previously only been attended by the nuclear family.

The first year Bob acquiesced he regretted it. The whole evening felt stilted and wrong to him.

"I felt like I had to watch every word," he remembers. "To make matters worse, the kids would look at me for every reaction. I had to school my face to keep it bland.

"My wife, bless her, knew what I was feeling. She would take my hand and squeeze it under the table and I would feel a little better physically."

Bob said he never felt his children were traitors. Instead, in his wisdom, he was proud that they were independent enough to think for themselves while still keeping a watchful eye on his reactions as they grew closer to their grandfather.

Inevitably the time did come where Bob had to function as the decision-making caregiver for his father. Don's bypass surgery had not been successful. His arteries were once again closing off.

They had had seven years of gradually forming a relationship before this happened. There were many visits and some Sunday dinners, although Bob still disliked sharing those precious times when his children were home from school. There were restaurant outings. And best of all, there was laughter.

Ultimately, when Don became ill Bob was able to go to him and help him make certain decisions about the time he had left. Bob became like most other Chadults—busy with his own life, yet involved with the care of his ill parent.

One day the two men were sitting quietly in the hospital room. Bob looked over at his father, who smiled weakly back at him. "Who knows," said the son, "maybe this was my mother's final gift to us all. We are together. I never thought it would be possible."

Sometimes when we deal in perceptions we can be very fortunate if we are challenged. After all, is it not possible that the impressions we garnered at very young ages could be inaccurate? We must allow some room for distortion in how we recall things.

Jeffrey still shakes his head when he sees his mother,

Marilyn, with his children. One day she was walking down the street with her two young granddaughters. A friend saw her with them and asked their ages.

The grandmother replied, "The doctor is four and the lawyer is six!"

This man searched his memory bank, but he could recall no time when his mother made little jokes about him. Life was somber. Life was important. He grew up in a nose-to-the-grindstone family.

That is why he finds his mother's lighter, happier behavior foreign. Chadults through the years have stood by in amazement watching their parents change personalities when dealing with grandchildren. The man was well aware of this possibility, but not until it became part of his life did he really believe it.

Betty, his wife, had heard stories about the dour upbringing her husband had experienced. His parents were strict people, no-nonsense people. Bend the rules even slightly and you were physically punished. She had heard so much that she felt trepidation when it was time to meet them before the wedding.

Indeed, they were not especially friendly to her. This relationship remained strained until she gave birth to her first daughter, who happened to be their first grandchild.

"It was like a mask had dropped from both of them— especially my mother-in-law," Betty says. "She couldn't hold my daughter enough or hug her enough. She stopped over all the time and brought little goodies for the baby."

Betty is an intelligent woman. She is able to see the trees *and* the forest. She started thinking about all the dreadful stories she had heard from her husband about his growing-up years. Despite his parents' firmness and inability to waver from a narrow path, they had given her husband a great deal. He was a moral man, a man of principle, a man upon whom she could count regardless of the problem. She smiled thinking he loved her fat and he loved her thin. Something really good must have been molded into him.

She saw these same strict people so loving and open with her daughter and then two years later with their next daughter.

Finally she decided it was time to talk to her husband, who was never pleased when his parents came to visit.

Betty sat down and shared her thoughts about his parents. She groped toward the idea that they had felt a strong sense of responsibility to impart values to their son. But now they felt free to love and enjoy without parenting responsibilities. Maybe her husband needed to begin to see them differently.

"After all," she pointed out, "they are going to get old, and how we choose to be part of their lives then will depend on how we build our relationship now."

Her husband could feel his own resistance to her words yet could not question their validity.

"It's such a hard thing for me," he said. "Can this be the father who used to be so angry? That guy who can't stop holding my daughter?

"Can this be my mother, who bawled me out every time a piece of paper fell on the floor—who now doesn't care when that same floor is crusted with mud brought in by her granddaughter? Which is really *them?*"

Betty had no answer except to tell him they were both seeing the same thing and it was beautiful.

Wise Chadults shake their heads and make no comments as they watch their parents play. They simply sit back and enjoy the scene. If they are lucky enough to have healthy parents the scene can often be riotous.

Cherish the time when they are able to enjoy the grandparent-grandchild relationship. Strive to spend as much time together as possible when your parent is still healthy enough to enjoy the children.

Take photographs of the different generations at play. Video home movies are excellent also. But it is the stills that the grandparents will hold on to and keep in safe boxes. If moving into a nursing home becomes necessary, they can find great comfort in pictures and showing them to other residents. The pictures say "I have a family. I have people who love me. Look at how I was able to play not so long ago."

When a Chadult begins to understand how much may be taken away from an aging parent—dignity, hope, future—he can best understand the importance of loving memories.

Often parent and child do not discuss their relationships and fears about the future. Mary, who lived in a nursing home, refused to share with her daughter, Beverly, how filled with gloom she was about the short time she had left to live. Despite much coaxing from Ann, a highly trained social worker, she kept her lips pursed tight.

One day during a one-on-one visit with Ann, the social worker, Mary finally explained her reasoning: "If I start complaining I'm afraid my daughter won't come. She won't bring her children. Then I am really a nobody here, just like those people who look like zombies sitting and never moving. I'd be a nobody."

The social worker fully understood the problem. One has status in a nursing home when one has visitors, just as an aging parent has status when neighbors know he or she is being cared for and seen by family members.

Although the world is no longer two-by-two for many of the elderly, there is still a sense that you are somebody when other people care. While this may not be the truth, it is certainly a perception some people cling to tenaciously.

Ann told Mary, "You seem like the sort of woman who would have raised a kind and caring daughter. I've met Beverly and I cannot imagine her abandoning you if she heard you share your fears."

"But I am not ready to risk it. I probably never will." Mary reached across the table and put her hand on Ann's arm. "I believe you can serve the function of hearing my fears. I want to give my family only good memories."

The social worker thought over what the woman had said. Was the risk worth it? Ultimately she decided Mary was not wrong; perhaps the risk *was* too great. She let things remain as Mary wished. Whenever Beverly stopped Ann to ask how her mother was doing, the social worker simply replied, "Well, look at her. She seems content. If you have any questions, ask her. She is extremely lucid."

Mary died about a year later, having never revealed her inner turmoil. According to the social worker, she died peacefully, surrounded by her loving family who spoke of her spirit and her spunk and her ability to adapt to whatever life had dealt her.

To this day Ann wonders if the daughter's knowing more about her mother's fears would have changed anything. The family appeared to be such a loving one.

But she learned from the experience. She no longer pushes people to purge themselves of their fears and dreads. Instead she always thinks of balance and always remembers the woman who had taught her its necessity.

Consider the old saying, "A son is a son until he takes a wife, but a daughter is a daughter the rest of her life." Is that always the case?

Certainly one young girl thought so. In a burst of the confidingness that children sometimes have, she told her mother, "I am nearer to you than I am to Papa." Her mother paused for a moment and then inquired, "Why, what do you mean, my dear?"

"Well," said the child, "I am your own little girl, but I am only related to Papa by marriage!"

There are indeed many daughters who feel a special bond with their mothers, and if all has moved swimmingly throughout the daughter's life, this bond continues until the mother dies.

It is rarely the case that she dislikes her father. She may, indeed, love him dearly. But the bonding is with her mother.

Certainly society assumes that should the mother become ill when she is older it is the daughter who will run to the doctor and see to her needs. This is so even though today many homes require two incomes, so that women have a work schedule to keep. And it is also the case where there are children who still require driving and parents' attendance at school functions.

There is nearly always a higher level of expectation placed on the daughter than on the son, and usually she will fall into line and accept whatever responsibility she sees must be met.

Cheryl works an average of sixty hours a week in an executive capacity for a major corporation. She has a husband and two high school–age children who were born in her mid-thirties. Her schedule is quite busy, but because she is an active, energetic person, she loves the challenge of keeping it all together.

But then a new problem appeared. Charlotte, her mother, who also was a prime example of strength and energy, had a stroke. She was completely incapacitated for months. Despite having nurses around the clock, the woman was belligerent and uncooperative unless her daughter was present.

Day care workers who tried as kindly as possible to help Charlotte with her medication and bathing and feeding were met with sealed lips, raging eyes, and a total unwillingness to help them help her. But when Cheryl arrived the woman would suddenly become more mellow. She would take her medication. She would allow herself to be bathed. She would eat a bit of food, although this was a slow and tedious process.

By the time all this was done it was late into the evening. Often Cheryl had not yet been home to see her own children and husband. She was frustrated and on the verge of exhaustion.

In anger, she called her brother, Elliot, and demanded that he come and help out.

"Hey, what are you getting mad at me for?" he asked. "I try to stop by every day, and she acts like I'm not there. She just wants you. That's what daughters are for, I guess." Cheryl was certain she detected a snippy tone in Elliot's voice.

Yet what was there for her to say? She certainly had not chosen to be placed in this position. But after all, she was the daughter, and what else was she to do?

Ultimately, Barry, her husband, intervened. He put his foot down when he saw her come through the door close to midnight knowing she had an eight o'clock meeting the following morning.

"I'm afraid this is it, honey," he said gently but firmly. "No more night forays to Mother's! We've gotten her the best care money can buy. You either trust the people you hired or you don't. I am going over there tomorrow and have a talk with her. I know she understands what is being said. She wouldn't be acting so stubborn if she didn't."

Cheryl plunked herself down on the couch, too weary even to take off her coat. This was some departure for her mild-mannered husband, who had always supported every endeavor she had undertaken. Now what was she supposed to do?

She laid her head back on the couch and closed her eyes. "The heck with it," she thought. "Let him do what he thinks is right. Elliot is no help and I can't go on like this too much longer."

The next day Charlotte was visited by a determined son-in-law. She had never seen him so unyielding. After all, one of Barry's nicest attributes was his willingness to go along with whatever the plans of the family might be. But here he was looking dark and angry.

He spent several hours with her and watched the nurse try to get pills down her throat. Charlotte resisted with all the strength she had left. He watched the nurse try to feed her and saw her spit the food at the woman.

That was when he snapped.

"This is ridiculous!" he yelled. "You are acting like an old fool! I've known you for forty years and respected you. I never thought I'd see you acting worse than my own daughter did during her terrible twos. I'm going to tell you this once and for all. Stop this foolishness and grow up!

"You want to get better. You want to go about your life. The doctor says there is no reason you can't if you cooperate. I've never seen such a display of disgusting childishness from a grown woman—especially you! If you want my respect back you're going to have to earn it."

Then he threw the clincher at her. "My wife—not your daughter, *my wife*—is in a state of near collapse from your demands. She will not be coming here every night from work any longer. She will create a schedule that is fair to both of you and to her family at home. You will not play this role with her any longer."

Charlotte sat defiant in her chair for some minutes. She looked her son-in-law directly in the eye and did not attempt to respond in any way. He never broke eye contact with her. In effect, he was going toe to toe with her, even though she was in a wheelchair.

Finally, she blinked first. She had not lost her ability to think, and she understood that this man was not only angry, he was serious about keeping her daughter away. "Well, more flies are caught with honey than with vinegar," she thought. Even more, was it possible she was being too demanding? She was so frightened by this sudden onslaught of incapacitation. She would have to learn to be a little smarter about her handling of her situation.

Barry saw her change in mood. He felt it. He spoke to the nurse. "Please try giving her the medicine again. I think we have straightened out a few things."

He was gratified when he saw his mother-in-law take her pills and then open her mouth to be fed.

"Cheryl will not be here tonight. She is too exhausted. But she will make some time to come by tomorrow. You're a tough old bird but I know you'll be fine. You've got plenty of fight left in you, that's for sure."

When he went home and told Cheryl what he had done she was angry at first. But after she saw he was determined she actually thanked him for acting as her protector in this situation. She sank gratefully into a bubble bath and slept the whole night through without a care. She felt no guilt. She felt no discomfort. She felt only the sense that her mother was being cared for—and, miracle of miracles, *so was she*.

This issue of a daughter's responsibility comes into play in another way as well. If a man is unmarried the assumption that he will take responsibility for the parent is usually not made. After all, he is a guy. He has work to do. He will be fumble-fingered if he tried to help out. That is rarely the case with a daughter.

When there is an unmarried daughter in the family, it is almost taken for granted that she will be the caregiver, regardless of how goal- and career-oriented she may be and how busy her life is.

Eileen, one such woman, was both a college professor and a psychologist in private practice. Despite her full schedule, which also included a varied and interesting social life, when her mother became ill, *she* was the one called regardless of whether it was day or night.

"There were times when I was furious," Eileen recalls. "I would be teaching or working with students on a project or seeing a private client and there would be a call that Mother needed to go to the doctor. She was ill. She needed to be taken to the hospital. She was upset. She was lonely. She needed some tender loving care.

"My family expected me to drop whatever I was doing and run to her side. I guess the rationale was my brother is a doctor and his wife is busy with their five little children. There were times when my resentment would nearly overwhelm me.

"But then I would remember what a great parent she had been. Now was my chance to say thank you. I needed to work at putting the unmarried-daughter issue behind me because that is one universal law that won't be changed for a long time to come, I'm afraid. I was not only her daughter. I was unmarried and therefore my time had less value, in the eyes of the family."

She said she once confronted her brother Irwin about this issue and he looked at her, surprised. "But of course that's true," he said. "I can't ask my wife to do everything for Mother, and I *am* far too busy to drop my practice and go running the way she would like me to. I guess you are the natural choice!"

To her credit Eileen left the room rather than fight over the issue. She felt that his indoctrination went so deep there was no possible way she could pry open his closed mind.

Demographic studies estimate that there will be thirteen million people aged sixty-five and older by the year 2010. Caring for them all is going to take a lot of planning and all the help that new technology can give.

But we live in a changing world. Many parents now carry beepers so their children can reach them regardless of where they are. This seems to offer comfort to both parents and offspring.

Frequently parents who live alone are perceived as being more vulnerable or in fact are more vulnerable. Their need to know there is a lifeline to their children is great, and the same beepers or pagers that meet the needs of parents with young children will probably become standard equipment for Chadults.

But here the comparison ends. Experts say the care of an aging parent and the inherent worry it creates generates far greater stress than child care because of its unpredictability. There is no way to anticipate life-altering falls, strokes, and heart attacks.

To add to the difficulty, many parents live a hundred or more miles away from their Chadults, which can mean racing down a highway or turnpike to get to the mother or father who is in distress.

These are not issues we can take lightly. The question is not whether we love our children more or our parents more. It is most important that we keep our perception and our priorities clear. As rational people we will generally go to the place where the fire needs putting out. If that place is home with our children, that is where we will place our energies. That is where we belong.

However, should we discover that our parents need our help, most of us will go that extra mile or one hundred miles to see that their needs are met.

While our base must always be in our own home, with our own children and family, we hope we will be able to make suitable arrangements for the care of our mothers and fathers. Those arrangements may be bringing them to our home for a time, seeing that they are comfortable in their own home, finding an establishment that will meet their needs, or some combination of all these things.

Most of all, we need to know where we are grounded. Cheryl, the hardworking executive, had lost that ability until Barry, her husband, brought the whole issue to the fore. How fortunate that she had a champion!

While, as we have seen, unmarried women have their own set of issues, there can be many variations when a group of offspring become Chadults and the mother or father becomes ill.

Some people say that life is one damned thing after another. But many Chadults would argue with this. They would instead say life is one damned thing over and over again. A case in point is the Marshall family.

The family consists of four siblings, two brothers and two sisters. All were college educated, and all had met their mates in college. Since all the mates were from out of state, each of the four Marshall siblings decided to move to a different part of the country after their marriages.

While their parents were appalled at each of the departures, they said nothing. But in their hearts and with each other they shared the dreadful fear of what would become of them if they became sick or widowed.

They had no way of knowing that their children had been quarreling fiercely amongst themselves long distance about just this issue. What *would* become of their parents now that they were left alone?

Sometimes the quarreling became almost silly squabbling. Marcy, one of the siblings, would even resort to saying, "I thought of moving first!"

Brian, her brother, might retort, "But look at my career here with my father-in-law!"

Mark, the other brother, might put in, "Well, I've already gotten my California license to practice law. I have clients!"

And Susan, the fourth sibling, would respond, "My husband is already established in Chicago. What do you expect us to do?"

Obviously, these young college graduates did care about their parents or there would have been no discussion over their having moved. But they had not yet reached the age when the fact that their parents would become old seemed a reality.

This fact generally doesn't hit home until the Chadult is forty or fifty—or even sixty, if the parent is healthy.

These Chadults had at least a vague sense that some thought should be given to their parents' future needs, but what those needs might be was extremely nebulous.

Certainly the Chadults had read articles on aging and seen movies that showed the plight of old people. These were not ignorant people. Yet watching their lovely mother leave for a party on the arm of her still-handsome husband did not equate with Jessica Tandy and Katharine Hepburn movies they had seen.

The four young people went off to their new lives but before they did they promised always to come "home" for Christmas. They shook on it, and for the first few years kept their promise. Christmas was always joyous and hectic for everyone. The parents cooked and planned and invited friends. Dinners were noisy and full of laughter.

When it was time for them to leave after the holidays, the departures were filled with haste and boisterousness and the promise to meet, same time, same place, next year.

They kept their commitment for about five years. Then gradually new factors crept in. Children were born and it became harder to travel. The young people who had settled in the north were tired of the cold and longed to take their long break in some sunny climate rather than in the northern state where their parents lived.

Yet they had made this commitment to one another and to their parents. The story is not unusual in that their best intentions began to fade with time.

Because physical distance separated them, the Chadults all continued to perceive their mother and father as youthful, vigorous, socially active people. This picture helped ease their discomfort about not coming "home" for Christmas each year.

Indeed, sometimes three and four years went by before one or another sibling visited with the parents. Still, when they would get together, they did not see the traces of inevitable aging.

Finally, one of those hallmark years came along. Mark, the eldest son, had his twentieth college class reunion. He called his parents, whom he hadn't seen for Christmas in about five years because his California law practice kept him tied to his office, and told them he and his family would indeed be there that Christmas holiday.

He also called the other siblings and begged them to make the effort so they could once again have a good old-fashioned reunion with one another. To his delight they all agreed to meet at home that year.

Meanwhile, their parents had gone about their lives, playing bridge and golfing and writing and phoning their children. Unfortunately, they were poor travelers and disliked being away from their own home. So they stayed put and lived their years together. They did not allow themselves to remember that five years had gone by since they had all been together with their children and grandchildren. That thought was just too depressing and it did not further their sense of well-being.

Mark was the first to notice that his parents had changed. His mother, while still quite attractive, had wrinkles around her eyes and mouth. Her posture, once the envy of his wife, was no longer as erect. Mark began to feel a vague discomfort as he watched his parents move a bit more slowly around their kitchen.

He did not call his siblings. Instead he waited for their arrival to see if they, too, noticed these little changes.

And each of them did. Suddenly the freedom and gaiety that had always been part of their vision of Christmas at home were no longer a given.

Why hadn't their parents written to tell them there were changes? Why didn't Dad say he had hurt his leg and limped a bit now? What else weren't they telling their children? Was money now becoming an issue? Did Mom and Dad have enough to meet their needs?

Late one evening, after the parents had gone to bed, the Chadults and their spouses sat in the living room and held the first of what would become a series of long family meetings and conference calls.

"I always pictured them younger and more vigorous."

"I always felt they could take care of themselves forever."

"I never thought about them aging."

"Well, what happens five years from now? Talk about aging!"

"We should be doing some deciding about all this."

"Maybe we should have them move to one of our cities. We can take care of them more easily from there."

"They'll never move!"

"We'll have to talk to them in the morning. I can't let this rest. They're not the kind of people who will come and cry to us, so we have got to step in and go to them."

But when the next morning came, the eight were loath to broach the subject. They kept looking to one another to see who would start the conversation.

Finally, Mrs. Marshall, who knew her children well, started laughing. "You're acting just the way you did when you were quite young and one of you smashed up the car. You all have that 'Who's going to break it to them?' look. What is going on here?"

Her husband, who had been glancing down at the paper, looked up and saw the same little-boy/girl-lost look on the faces of his offspring and their spouses. He lit a cigarette and after taking a deep puff reiterated his wife's question: "Yes, what *is* going on here?"

There was silence at the table. The siblings looked at one another. Finally, they all looked at Mark, their eldest brother, and waited for him to speak. He did.

"This is really awkward, Dad, Mom. It's just that we all haven't seen you for a few years and all of us noticed changes. Changes in both of you."

"Why, whatever do you mean?" asked his mother.

Mark gritted his teeth. This was not going to be easy.

"Well, we see the sort of changes that make us feel a bit concerned about you. Oh, Dad's using that cane now and then. You're a little slower in the kitchen. Things like that."

"We don't mean to say we think you're old," said Marcy, trying to jump in to Mark's rescue.

"Well, then, dear, what *are* you trying to say?"

Again, a silence descended on the room.

Mr. Marshall looked over at Mark. "Come on, son, we're not ogres. You've always felt free to talk to us about anything. If you have a problem, let Mom and me help if we can."

"Well, you see, Dad, what we're concerned about is you and Mom. Don't get me wrong—you're both doing great. But we're concerned about what if something happens. All of us are so far away."

"Why, how thoughtful of you. All of you. It's something Dad and I think about a great deal."

"Have you come up with any conclusions? Any ideas?"

"Well, as long as we have each other things don't seem as immediate. What we are concerned about is if something happens to one of us."

Susan, the youngest daughter, looked at her mother intently. "Have you thought about any alternatives if that should happen? You know this is very painful to even talk about, but maybe we need to."

Her mother shook her head. "Every time one of us comes up with a suggestion the other seems to nix it. So, so far no alternatives."

Mark looked over at his wife and she nodded almost imperceptibly—but not quite imperceptibly enough for her mother-in-law to miss it. "We were wondering if you would consider coming out to California and living near us. That way you would have some family."

The other Chadults chimed in with similar offers.

"We talked about that and it's hard at our age to think of pulling up stakes and making new friends. While it would be marvelous to know we can call a son or daughter should we become ill, you all have your own lives just as we have ours. We still have our friends and social engagements. No, as long as we are able, I don't think that that would be a good solution."

Her husband nodded. "I do want to thank you for your concern. It helps us should we have to make a major decision to know we are welcome and wanted. I do promise we will think further and let you all know what we decide."

"Now, about all this pile of breakfast. Let's dig in!"

There was relief in the air. A major inaccurate perception had been dispelled. These parents *had* been thinking about their aging. While nothing would be resolved during this trip, all ten people at the table knew a process had begun.

The Chadults felt comfortable. They knew their parents to be orderly, methodical people, and they were assured that things would be thought out and explored, and important decisions would be made with care.

There is a further moral to this story. Chadults often, though certainly not always, underestimate the people who raised them. The Marshalls demonstrated this. Just because someone is getting on in years does not mean they have lost their ability to see things objectively. After all, the parents are the most interested parties. If their mental faculties are intact, they can see the seriousness of making decisions that will affect the rest of their lives.

When Chadults who are genuinely concerned feel that dreaded moment has come when "the conversation about the future" is inevitable, they would be wise to remember the story of a world-famous speaker.

Once his son was visiting and saw his father preparing a speech.

"Dad, do you still have to prepare for a speech after all this time? Don't you know what you will say?"

"My son," answered the orator, "I don't have to prepare what I will say, but I do have to prepare what I will *not* say!"

Tact and delicacy can't but be helpful when the time comes for the all-important conversation. It doesn't have to be—and shouldn't be—handled bluntly, with all the cards on the table and quick-fix solutions at the ready, if there is no emergency. When families can take their time they will see the benefits of planning.

Of course, if there is a sudden illness, sometimes Chadults are left with no alternative but bluntness. They cannot do anything but tell it like it is. Time is of the essence in these situations. If Father needs a nursing home and Mother is homebound she certainly cannot be left alone.

Arrangements may have to be made quickly. This is especially difficult when children live out of town. Should the parents remain at home? Should they move to the Chadult's city? How hard it is to have to make such decisions in a matter of days!

But if any Chadult has it within his or her power to sit and talk about this difficult topic in a firm and orderly manner, without being dictatorial, the need to do so is great.

To have a plan can be the greatest comfort to everyone involved—and that includes parents who might initially have been reluctant to look down the unpleasant road of illness and infirmity that many elderly people have to face.

There is an old saying that when we are twenty we plan what we will do at forty, but when we reach sixty or thereabouts we plan what we're going to do after breakfast.

It's all in the perception.

Perception also plays a major role in how Chadults see the fact of "obligation."

It is a word that is two-sided.

All too often Chadults see their interaction with their aging parents as a duty, an obligation.

While most Chadults recognize they will in some way *have* to interact with their aging parents, the issue to consider is how they see their adult children's role. What do they want it to be?

When what is done is done with a mean spirit, the recipient can always tell. Make no mistake about that. It's hard to be in a position where one needs help and must accept it with a smile regardless of how grudgingly it is given!

It is equally hard to be in the position of *having* to help without any desire to do so. Giving help grudgingly is uncomfortable for the Chadult as well.

That is the kind of obligation that is negative. Help must be given, but only out of a sense of responsibility.

One of the intangible factors in the parent–child relationship is the hard fact that no vows are ever exchanged. No formal commitment is ever made. While there is a given that a person who brings a child into the world owes it nurturing and a warm safe place in which to live, there is no formal commitment on the other end.

Your child does not take any vow to care for you or love you or protect you. While this may sound harsh it is nevertheless true.

What a Chadult gives is a gift. Chadults, for the most part, know this at some level. How generous or kind they choose to be is very much up to them.

Certainly Chadults can be victimized by guilt-tripping. It is a technique used frequently by parents who must get their needs met. The consequence of such a tactic, however, is not always so pleasant: physical needs may be met, but warm fuzzies are absent. Parents need those warm fuzzies as much as young children and Chadults do. A kind word, a gentle stroke on the arm can strengthen the will to go on in someone who is saddened by his plight in life.

Guilt-tripping can certainly be frustrating to a Chadult who feels she has done and given as much as she wants to or can. Then she may feel the need to move to another stage. She makes herself less available: "Sorry, Mom. I'm just too busy today."

And, yes, there is even that technique that we usually hear about in relation to very difficult teenagers: "Toughlove."

Barry demonstrated Toughlove when he took a no-nonsense approach with his mother-in-law. When he told Charlotte that her daughter would no longer be at her beck and call, she knew he meant it. When he insisted she take hold of her conduct toward her nurses, he demonstrated Toughlove. Had she not been wise enough to hear him clearly, she might well have been in danger of losing positive contact with her daughter.

Any number of Chadults have resorted to just this type of behavior in order to make "no" stick, in order to make certain their own lives are not trampled and turned upside down by unreasonable demands. Toughlove is most common when the parent is under the strong impression that he or she is "owed" certain things.

Perhaps in all the aging process there is nothing that causes more damage to a relationship between parents and children than this "obligation" hang-up.

Some aging parents remind their Chadults that they have obligations. That type of obligation implies guilt. It implies that the Chadult's needs are not as important as the parent's. Obligation presented this way brings resentment and anger. There is very little in this that is positive. All those building blocks that needed to be put in place over the years in order to have a more loving aging time obviously did not come together.

Chadults, most of whom are good and decent people, feel very uncomfortable when they must do without a loving heart.

The best they can offer is to accommodate all the different pullings they feel. Certainly the squeaky wheel gets the most attention. But aging parents must understand they pay a price. That price can be high when things are not given willingly. When the atmosphere is filled with hostility and anger, everyone feels it.

Certainly the person in need, the aging parent, if alert at all, cannot miss the signals. The Chadult and his family arrive for Sunday dinner. The car door slams a little harder than necessary. "Well, what do you want to drink?" "Look, we made plans for dinner this evening so we'll sit with you while you eat and then we're off." Annoyance seeps through every sound that comes from behind the gritted teeth.

Yet despite all these negative attitudes and vibrations, Mother will pretend to be oblivious. She will ignore her daughter-in-law's impatience. She will ignore her grandson's pulling at her Chadult son's arm.

She does need these people. She is alone. But she also needs to see that it is possible to fill her Sunday evening with other people if this is the reception she is getting from her family. Her self-esteem can keep her healthy and even alive, according to many medical experts. But how to make her understand this?

On the other hand, Sunday is the last time to stretch out and take it easy before yet another week of work and industrious activity begins for the Chadult.

Some families take Mother to brunch or a three o'clock dinner. But that still leaves her with a long evening ahead, and probably a long week as well. Many parents recognize this and show their resentment at being left behind so early in the day. It does not help them get what they most want: the *loving* attention of their children.

That is why is might be very helpful to set a plan with some friends or neighbors who are faced with the same situation. Together, perhaps, you can help guide Mom or Dad to an activity that will take place in alternating homes later in the day. This plan can certainly be put in place by the Chadult, and it makes Mom even more attractive if she is busier and hence less available.

This is a sad but often true fact of life.

Without question there is always the chance that though you have led the horse to water you can't make her drink. But if you have entertained Mom for some portion of Sunday and tried to make arrangements for the rest of the day, you can feel some relief from the dreaded "obligation" factor.

On the other hand, there are some beautiful "obligation" stories. These obligations are the ones that are handled with great love and tenderness, as the Chadult looks for an opportunity to repay. "Thank you" seems so inadequate for a whole life of being on this earth, a life filled with an abundance of love and concern and warmth.

Paula was just such a mother. She filled her life with bringing peace and joy to her son and daughter and husband. She was a gentle woman, yet fierce as a lioness if her cubs were attacked.

In her later years she developed a fatal form of cancer. Her children, both grown and married, wanted to make her last year as meaningful as possible.

Since money was not a barrier the daughter, Pauline, who lived in the same town, moved into the same condominium complex as her mother.

"That way, if she needed me, I was there," Pauline says. "I am blessed with a husband who loved me enough to understand that this was my time to give back all I had been given. He understood that my time to do so was limited. My mother's life was nearly over."

Pauline says there were many nights her mother could not sleep. Her mother was in pain but did not want to spend her remaining year drugged and unable to think. She was completely alert. Pauline told her mother when those bad nights occurred to simply call and she would walk across the road and visit with her.

"We would end up playing Scrabble. Both of us competed fiercely and even though the call would come at five in the morning, we would go on until she finally felt like sleeping. I would walk her to her bedroom and tuck her in and kiss her and tell her how much I loved her."

Pauline would then go home and catnap. "Certainly I would be tired. But I knew we only had about a year. There would be plenty of time after that for me to rest."

Pauline's brother, George, lived halfway across the country. He flew in every other weekend because he wanted to spend time with his mother whom he loved dearly.

Since his sister was the primary caregiver, George used to beg Pauline to take a break, to go away for a weekend with her husband. He could certainly manage caring for their mother unaided.

But Pauline declined. She loved her brother very much and saw his concern for both of them. But, she insisted, "when you're here like this it makes me feel like we're a family, all living in one place again. Why would I leave you and not visit during this special time?"

Their mother saw only love and tenderness for her and had the great satisfaction of knowing that when she was dead the bond between sister and brother would remain strong and loving.

"At the end, it gave her great peace. She died at home. We were all in her room holding hands with her and one another. It was a death watch and a love-in at the same time," Pauline observed.

She says she and her brother had been fortunate in that her mother had been farsighted. She knew that at some point down the road illness was a real possibility, and before she became ill she had written each of her children a letter expressing her wishes.

"When I got the letter I was very upset," Pauline remembers. "What was a hale and hearty sixty-year-old woman doing thinking about such things? But, like the wonderful mother she was, she gave us a road map of how she wanted to be handled. She never asked me to move my residence, of course; that was my own decision. But she didn't want to be knocked out with painkillers. It was one of her fears about wasted time. Having that letter gave us our assurance that we were returning in kind all that she had given us."

This same type of positive obligation affected the Marshall family we met earlier.

Their concern was how best to help their parents with a given set of circumstances. They wanted to allow them as much dignity and as much independence as possible. And, best of all, they were able to act as a family unit.

It is said that good heredity deals you a fine hand of cards, and a loving environment teaches you to play the hand well.

Perception always matters. If the Chadult is willing to be open-minded and perhaps ask *why* when he was young certain things were done the way they were, this perception may take on new dimensions. In this present era, it's useful to keep in mind that fifty or sixty years ago things might have been handled in a different manner because there was less focus on and discussion about child-raising. Sometimes when parents say, "I did it for your own good," they genuinely mean it. They believe they acted in your interests.

Having a long talk with the parent from whom you feel distanced can sometimes be valuable. But remember, the parent has little ability to change her behavior of the past. If *you* believe you will feel more comfortable in having said your piece, then it serves a purpose . . . especially if you can go forward with kindness after you are through.

Obligations are in the eyes of the beholder. One perceives them as either an onerous duty or an act of love. If you look at your parents as the people who brought you life, perhaps that will help you see the positive side of obligation. It might enable you to act more lovingly.

Ultimately, this will give you greater peace when they die. This is what makes a loving obligation the more desirable.

Remember, love doesn't make the world go round. Love is what makes the ride worthwhile.

Chapter 4

THE

TIME FOR

DECISIONS

◇

The great majority of us are required to
live a life of constant duplicity. Your
health is bound to be affected if, day
after day, you say the opposite of what
you feel, if you grovel before what you
dislike, and rejoice at what brings you
nothing but misfortune.

—Boris Pasternak

Once a peasant traveled on foot along a red clay back road in his native Russia. His feet began to ache from walking so long and far, and he started to pray: "Oh, Lord, if I only had an animal to ride!"

No sooner were these words out of his mouth than a rough-looking farmer came trotting along on a donkey. The donkey he rode had just given birth.

"Here, you," ordered the farmer, cracking his whip, "take this baby donkey on your shoulders and carry it for me!"

The peasant was frightened of the rough man and did as he was ordered. He trudged behind the farmer, carrying the small donkey on his shoulders.

As he staggered along, bent nearly double from the weight of his burden, he said to himself, "Truly, my prayer has been fulfilled! I did not express myself clearly enough when I prayed for help. I should have stipulated that I wished to have an animal for *me* to ride—not one to ride me!"

All too often Chadults find themselves in the same situation. Mother or father, on whom the Chadult once depended, is now saying, "I need help." But what *is* help?

Specificity can clear the air as nothing else will. Yet few conversations in a Chadult's life will prove more difficult. How do you sit down with people who are dressed for golf or planning a trip and say, "Now, we've got to look down the road. You may not be tomorrow where you are physically today." Who wants to hear this? Who wants to say this?

How can you introduce the topic of the inevitable prognosis of aging when you know it will replace the bright sparkle in your mother's eyes with the fear that probably already lurks in the back of her mind?

The question that always seems so unanswerable is why parents are willing to discuss stocks and wills and inheritances more freely. Perhaps they are able to remove themselves. After all, they are talking about when they are dead.

Have we reached a time and place in our world where it is better and easier to talk about dying than about aging?

Helen would answer that question with a resounding yes.

She is in her early seventies and still plays cards and bingo and meets friends for lunch. She likes to cook and frequently has small dinner parties in her senior apartment.

One evening at just such a dinner party, two of her friends, Myrna and Joyce, both widowed, were sharing their experiences in a role that was several years old for both of them. They agreed: "Despite my husband's faults I sure would like him back. It's lonely being a widow."

These women still planned short trips for the summer; their conversation was animated, and there was a lot of laughter.

But they had to deal with pain and loneliness and watching their money. Myrna had a son whose marriage was ending, which added to her worries. She cared for her daughter-in-law and adored her grandchildren. She feared she would no longer have easy access to them. Their future was high on her list of concerns.

"But I've lived long enough to know that anything I say won't make any difference anyhow," she said. "So I do what we all do. Live for now and enjoy what I can and try to see no evil and hear no evil and speak no evil."

Her dinner companions nodded. For each, in her own way, had been faced with a similar choice.

They had discovered that staying out of harm's way was a safe and wise way of life. And the proof of this was evident in how they were still able to enjoy what life had to offer them.

Could we look at this picture and say these women were behaving not like human beings but like ostriches hiding their heads in the sand? Possibly. But if that is what an ostrich must do to survive, then it is not all bad. The species is not extinct.

Perhaps another reason death is easier for Chadults and their parents to discuss than the long tunnel of illness and aging is because, like this group of widows, they have stared in the face of death and seen they could go on. Aging and deterioration do not offer the same comfort.

Wilbert, an octogenarian who now resides in a nursing

home and is wheelchair-bound, describes his circumstances well: "I was a fine, strapping young man. I worked hard and built an excellent business. I helped raise fine children. All I ever saw in my life was a great sense of going forward on to the next plateau, the next level—whether that was in business or seeing my children graduate from college or becoming a grandfather and even a great-grandfather. Everything was going forward. That was how my mind was geared, and you know what? I liked it! I liked it a lot!

"I provided for my family and myself financially. When my wife died I hired a housekeeper and kept myself busy."

Asked if he had ever thought about these later years and the possibility of not being well physically, he raises his hand in a gesture of despair.

"If I did, I sure pushed it back in my mind. I didn't want to think about it. How does a healthy, vigorous man allow himself to picture being like this?" He gestures around the wheelchair and the visiting lounge of the nursing home. "This is what happens to those old people they make movies about. It doesn't happen to strong, active men like myself!"

But it *did* happen to him, and it happens to endless numbers of people like him.

Many of them are not isolated. They have family members who love them, who care about their well-being and are perhaps even overprotective. Maybe it is time to open the closet and look squarely at the facts:

- If we live we will age
- Medicine will keep us alive longer
- We will probably need an illness portfolio, detailing our wishes, before we need a stock portfolio
- Not discussing these truths as a family can be harmful to the unit as a whole. This is especially true when

parents have not abrogated their positions but have
remained parents even as their children became
Chadults

Timidity can overtake even the most responsible Chadult
when he or she is faced with a parent who has always functioned at a high level. Such parents have raised their children
to believe that parents sit on Olympus and are the masters of
all they survey.

When that is the case, how does the Chadult broach the
topic of the parent's wishes should he or she become ill?

It is necessary to talk with Mom and Dad about their
wishes while they are alert. Without question, this is a most
difficult topic to bring up. No one likes to look down the road
at the likelihood that things will not be at least as good as they
are today but will in fact probably be worse.

The most fortunate Chadults are those with pragmatic parents who see what is coming and have the kind of abundant
love that allows them to make certain their adult children do
not have to make uninformed decisions—uninformed, that is,
about what the parent might wish.

Lawrence had been widowed less than a year. He lived in
the apartment he had shared with his wife and found that he
still automatically wanted to turn to her and ask her advice.
When he realized he was doing this, he began making it a
habit to call his daughter.

When he saw after yet another year had gone by that
nothing had dramatically changed—that he still automatically
wanted his wife's input, and that he was calling up his daughter more and more—he decided that the long road ahead did
not bode well for him. He was a man in his seventies, and
while he did socialize with women, he had no interest in
remarriage.

One day he sat down at his desk and in a thoughtful and precise manner wrote out his wishes. He did not do what the peasant trudging down the road did, with vague hopes for an easier way. He spelled out just what he wanted.

He wanted to be kept in his home as long as possible.

Although he would have liked to contribute to his grandchildren's college and other such "luxuries," he preferred that whatever money he had accrued be used for his care at home.

Should it become evident that he was no longer able to remain in his apartment, he wanted his children to sort through his possessions. He designated specific antique pieces for each of his three daughters, two of whom lived out of town.

After all avenues for his home care had been exhausted he wished to be placed in a nursing home. He had been investigating and found one that contained many people of his ethnic background.

He did not wish to be kept alive on machinery should he be found in that situation. He also stated funeral and burial wishes.

When his children saw the document there was some argument. "But we can take you in. You can live with us. Why didn't you talk with us about all this? We didn't know how you were feeling."

He stopped them all. In the same soft-spoken but purposeful manner he had employed all his life in dealing with his family, he explained these wishes were not the whim of a moment, but part of a well-thought-out plan. He expected his Chadults to honor them because he wanted the comfort of knowing there would be dignity—as well as the respect of his family—allowed him in his final years, just as there had always been.

This man was unlike the many people described by Pasternak. There was no duplicity. It would perhaps have been easier for the moment had he said yes, certainly, to each child who came up with a new life plan for him.

But in the end he would have left great confusion. "But Dad said" would have gone ringing from household to household. The room for misinterpretation would have been great, and such misinterpretation could have led to real conflict between his children, something he wished to avoid.

But Lawrence was more the exception than the rule. He was obviously a goal-oriented man, someone who saw his options, laid out his tasks, and set about solving the problems that could arise. Because he was this type of person he was able to hold and command the respect of his family, respect that can be hard to keep as people age.

Although his line of communication with his children was very open and calls were made back and forth quite freely, he kept a part of himself to himself, and in some way his self-sufficiency and certainty of direction made him more attractive and desirable to his children. They sought him as much as he sought them.

There is a story about a mother who gave her college-bound son two neckties as a going-away present. When he came home on a visit he wore one of the ties to let her see his appreciation of her gift.

The mother took one look at the tie and asked unhappily, "What's the matter? Didn't you like the other one I gave you?"

Unfortunately, far too many Chadults are caught up in this type of interaction, where there is no getting it right, rather than that of the father with his clearly laid plans.

Most parents, caught in their fear of aging and their denial that it is happening and that death is inevitable, work very assiduously at avoiding the issues. But again, ironically, the more we seek to avoid the more difficulty we may have when avoiding the issues becomes impossible.

Such avoidance can affect one's health. Parents may ignore a cough or pay no attention to a slight dizziness. They force themselves to ignore ignore ignore the symptoms that cry out for doctoring. Often, by the time their adult children fully understand that Mother is really unwell, it is too late to do much to help her.

This, of course, is the opposite of the parent who is constantly calling the doctor, demanding rides to his office, and being told time and again there is nothing wrong.

The difficulty of dealing with this second type of mother or father is to know when to take them seriously. How does even a Chadult who grew up in a home with these people know when to believe there is really a problem?

Far too often the Chadult discussing his mother will attach the label "hypochondriac" to her. He will complain that everything seems to be a huge "final" ailment until Mother is taken to the doctor and told it's only gas.

But when you are old and afraid, there is no such thing as "only." Each episode, each body change, each time you forget something reminds you that you are aging and becoming frail.

Sometimes, in order for a Chadult to take charge of her parent's situation, she must first take charge of her own feelings.

Take a deep breath.

Count to ten.

Force yourself to recall something good from your childhood—even if it's the number of times you cried out at night that you were sick when in fact there was nothing really wrong but fear of the dark. Remember how your mother held you and rocked you until you were comforted.

Try to organize a schedule that *does* allow time for your parents. While they will probably always feel it is not enough, they should not have to beg for some attention.

Use that time for appointments or marketing. Taking care of necessities in an orderly manner alleviates discomfort for the parent and frustration on the part of the Chadult about what must be done.

Allow yourself to enjoy your mother and father. Certainly they will have habits—probably ones that have caused you lifelong annoyance—that continue to grind at you. But surely they must have some redeeming qualities. You are a product of what they were capable of producing!

Laugh with them. Let them relive stories they have told a hundred times. Enjoy their enjoyment. It may not be your idea of pleasure, but it is theirs, and you may find *that* actually brings you pleasure.

In other words, use the same kindness and respect with your parents that you would display to a stranger. Kindness is much more productive than outbursts of temper and frustration. Indeed, it can be hard to keep kindness up at times. It is irritating for the Chadult who has her whole day planned out to get that panicky call in the morning saying, "I'm sick and the doctor will see me at two o'clock."

It is hard to swallow the annoyance of having to cancel a bridge game, a tennis lesson, a college class.

But few Chadults have not experienced this many times. The issue is how to handle it. Certainly snapping at Mother will not change her pattern. She is panicked and will do what she needs to do to help herself. Even if she is not always alert, even if she is sometimes a bit fuzzy around the edges, her instinct to survive remains strong. Yes, even when she tells you she wishes she were dead, she probably doesn't mean it. This may be *her* cry in the night and *her* fear of the dark.

The simplest thing you can do to help is to initiate an honest conversation. Let her know how much you appreciate all she did in raising you. The time she spent doing things that interested you. The times she went out of her way to make your life pleasant and fun and perhaps a bit easier during your turbulent teen years.

Then point out that just as her life was so crammed full during those years, yours is crammed full now. Give her a schedule of your daily chores and plans that is as detailed as possible. Let her see on paper what your days consist of. Tell her things do come up that are unexpected. She will already know you have a passion for bridge. Let her know occasionally you are asked to sit in on a game unexpectedly or you are asked to be someone's tennis partner. But you will do the best you can to accommodate her doctor appointments if she will promise to look at your schedule when making them.

This sounds logical, doesn't it? It all sounds as if it should be simple and no problem for either of you. But usually when Mother gets panicky your carefully prepared schedule goes out the window.

You are stuck with your anger and annoyance and—face it—unwillingness to have anything to do with hypochondria.

The problem can be that sometime it won't be hypochondria. Sometime she truly will be ill. How will you know when it's the real thing? Perhaps she will call, panicked because she's dizzy, and you will say, "Not today, Mom, I have a game," only to find out later that she had a mild stroke that did indeed need medical attention.

You may then be left feeling like a bad, selfish person who has always taken and never given back. Most likely you will forget all the kind things you have done for her as you see her lying in her hospital bed. You see your mother, and how little she looks lying there. How pitifully small.

The question is asked time and time again: When do I really step in? Am I taking away a precious independence by becoming my parent's parent? Am I being lax as a daughter by not intervening?

Further, when a Chadult finds herself on this threshold, she may realize she cannot bear to lose her role as child. That feeling cannot be ignored. As long as you can retain even the slightest vestiges of the familiar parent-child relationship, you can feel somewhat safe. Your parents are the ones you can turn to and say, "Do you remember . . . ?" That is one of life's most precious links. It is the bridge between our youth and the here-and-now. Since life is lived in a continuum and not in fits and starts, that bridge is precious to most Chadults. And it is indeed important to keep alive the memories of our nurtured and secure lives as youngsters.

Our hurt and disillusionment begin to grow when we turn as we always have to Mom or Dad and they don't remember that all-important incident in our lives. For many Chadults this is the time when we need to straighten our shoulders and acknowledge that things are not as they were before and never, except at intervals, will be again.

But how do we deal with this new information? Certainly if we have siblings we can turn to them and continue to share the stories with them.

We can tell our spouse, who probably has some interest in our past and our youth.

We can share stories with our children. They, probably most of all, will be interested, because not only are you revealing yourself to them during your most vulnerable growing-up years, you are also giving them new family insights. If told well, these stories can build yet another bridge—a three-generational span!

Don't let the memories die. Don't let the stories die. They are your history bank—the continuum of your life—and they serve a real purpose, because no one is without a history.

While it is necessary to live in the present, we are the sum total of our experiences. Those experiences made us the people we have become. Just as it is valuable to study history in school to learn how our civilization has evolved to this point, so it is necessary to understand how we have evolved as individuals.

There is an irony in all this that most Chadults push away or refuse to acknowledge. Regardless of how old we are, we almost always have unfinished business. Whether that business was receiving or not receiving Mom's approval or Mom's love, whether Mom favored a sister or brother over us, that freeway of memory may have some rough patches.

Estrangement can heighten your questioning about when and where you should step in as your parents age. Just seeing them in a weakened condition can be frightening and intimidating, even for an accomplished, high-powered Chadult.

Many Chadults carry an unspoken hope that somehow, magically, all the old hurt will not merely disappear but will be resolved. Yet, when you start your dialogue and try to clear up old issues, Mom and Dad don't seem to focus on how important these issues were and are to you.

You may face them with past hurts about which you still feel passionately, and they just look at you knowing their lives are nearly over.

Where is the meeting point?

Some Chadults feel reluctant to step in and make decisions precisely because of these unresolved issues.

"Am I doing it from proper motivations?"

"Am I being punitive?"

"How do truly loving children behave in this situation?"

"If I call the doctor, will Mom really want my brother and not me there with her?"

"But whenever I call my brother about her he is busy, even though she loved him more."

And so the line of questioning goes, never ending unless the Chadult does some true soul-searching or seeks therapy.

Most people feel a certain timidity about intervening in someone else's life even if that person is their own parent. How much greater the uncertainty becomes when that intervention means life-changing alterations!

The idea that these people raised you and now you are reversing *everything* is so daunting that some Chadults are never able to take control. They will allow themselves to be led by doctors and social workers and some health-care givers. At the back of their minds is always the thought that they personally never really made the decision. Others helped. This can be especially reassuring to those who are somewhat timid, or uncomfortable in the role of taking care of their parents.

Sometimes taking charge is a reaction rather than an action. We see something that is not right. We jump in and supply the remedy. Many Chadults learn to their displeasure and dismay that they might have been wiser to think and plan and test the waters before diving headlong into a new role.

Kathy and her mother had played bingo once a week for years. Both women would look forward to the evening spent together. Mom would stop at Kathy's and visit with her teenaged grandchildren, then the two women would go out to dinner and play late into the evening.

"I think it began so slowly that I didn't even notice," Kathy says. "Not until now when I think back. It just seemed to happen so smoothly. So naturally. One night as we were driving to play I noticed Mom was gripping the steering wheel very hard and her neck was leaning forward in a tense position.

"I asked her why she was driving like that and she said it was really nothing, just that she seemed to need a little more concentration when she drove at night.

"The next week I called her and told her I would pick her up, and she seemed almost grateful. She didn't argue about not seeing the kids or anything."

As she thinks back on this seemingly small occurrence, Kathy believes the decision for her to drive began the mother-daughter role reversal. This role change would last for the remainder of Kathy's mother's life.

What Kathy believes created the difficulties that followed was the women's failure to have an honest dialogue.

"I made a decision," she says. She was obviously wise in not wishing her mother to drive at night if it could be stressful—indeed, potentially hazardous. "But I never asked how she felt about it. She sounded, and probably *was,* relieved. But as two adults we should have had a discussion."

As time went on, Kathy saw more and more of her mother's infirmities. There were occasions such as the time Kathy had planned an afternoon out with friends and her mother called to say she had forgotten that she had an appointment with her cardiologist at two o'clock. When this sort of thing happened, Kathy would have to cancel her plans. She would become angry. Finally she began keeping a calendar of her mother's appointments and planning her life around them.

"My husband, Jason, realized what was happening and he became very angry. He worked hard so that I would not have to work outside the home, and here I was working around my mother and not my husband and kids.

"I made the mistake of letting him see how frustrated I was one day when I was asked to play pinochle. I told my friend to hold the phone while I went to check my mother's appointment calendar and he heard me. I was already irritated because I had to do that. I resented the daylights out of these intrusions. Now, to add to that, my husband was very angry.

"I would get furious enough sometimes that it would show in my driving and my mother would ask what was wrong. I would snap at her and tell her to be quiet. It got to the point where there was nothing she could say or do that I did not resent. I started yelling at her and reminding her of every hateful thing I could remember from my childhood. I didn't care that she cried."

Finally Kathy and Jason went to see a therapist, a social worker who dealt often with problems concerning aging parents. Kathy came to see that she was not only experiencing resentment, but also facing the inevitability of her mother's death and her own sense of helplessness and feeling of abandonment by the parent she loved.

Many—if not all—Chadults are caught in this trying situation. They recall all that was done for them and feel the need to do for their own families as well as for their parents.

If a Chadult does things for Mom that are loving and kind, then that is indeed the positive fulfillment of an obligation that will always be appreciated and remembered by everyone concerned.

If, however, she does things out of a sense of duty alone, an indescribable hurt may be felt not only by the parent, who feels burdensome and useless and questions why she has been allowed to live so long, but also by the Chadult, who is ashamed of not feeling the loving-kindness toward Mom that so many of her dear friends express about their own parents.

As in all things that are important in life, we must recognize the need for balance. If we can live in a positive manner and see obligation as an act of love and caring, then we will be the better and healthier for it. We will see ourselves in the role of caregiver from its most positive perspective, and that can make our sense of obligation one of peace.

As we find resolution in one aspect of our lives, we can face the next one regarding our parent with a little more ease. If we can discover a formula to help us resolve aspects of our relationship, it can be used repeatedly. It is when our entire relationship seems confused that we find ourselves unable to make appropriate decisions about how to handle new situations.

Finding peace can give us a beautiful sense of obligation and the comfort of knowing that we are dealing appropriately with our parents.

There once was a rabbi who traveled by train to visit his daughter who lived in the city.

Since smoking was allowed in his particular car, he lit a cigarette. A young man seated next to him began grumbling.

"The smell of that cigarette is disgusting," he said.

The rabbi apologized. "I didn't know you disliked the smell of smoke. I'll put out my cigarette."

The other passengers in the car looked on in amazement. "What is that man doing in this car if he doesn't like the smell of smoke?" they asked one another. "He should move to a nonsmoking compartment!"

A few minutes later the same young man complained about the cold. "I can't stand sitting next to this man. I'm freezing and the window is open."

"I'm sorry, sir," said the rabbi. "I wasn't the one who opened the window, but I'll be glad to close it," and he did so.

The fellow passengers were amazed at the kindness with which the impressive-looking old man treated the young man. He seemed to indulge him as if he were a child.

When the train arrived at its destination, the station platform was packed with people who had come to welcome the rabbi. As soon as he got off the train he was surrounded by the throng.

"Welcome! Welcome!" could be heard around the platform.

The young man saw the fervor of the reception and asked his fellow passengers who the man was.

"Don't you know? He is the great rabbi of his community."

The young man felt sick and slunk away, but he first asked if anyone knew where the great rabbi was staying.

He was told the rabbi was staying with his son-in-law, himself a rabbi of some repute in the community to which they had come.

The young man went to his inn. He tried to eat but the food caught in his throat. He went to his room to lie down but he couldn't find rest. That entire night he lay sleepless. What had he done?

He could barely wait until it was daylight before finding the son-in-law's home. The rabbi with whom he had traveled greeted him graciously.

"Have a seat. How are you feeling? Do you like your lodging? What do you think of this great big city?"

The young man remained standing and suddenly burst into tears. "Rabbi, please forgive me. . . . I didn't know . . ."

"Sit down and relax," the rabbi told him. He assured the young man he was not angry. He said he understood that a young man is likely to let his emotions get away from him. "After all, we are only human. People learn from their mistakes."

The young man's eyes lit up. He listened to everything the rabbi told him and promised that he would be considerate of other people from then on.

As he got up to leave the rabbi stopped him. "Would you mind telling me why you came to this city? Do you have family here?"

"No, sir. I have no one here. I am newly married and I am looking for a position as a teacher at the rabbinical college in this city."

"Well, if that's so, I can help you. My son-in-law can help you meet the people you must talk with. Let's ask him now."

The rabbi led the young man to the son-in-law's study and explained what he hoped to accomplish.

The son-in-law, a great scholar, tested the young man on the spot but found that he was not of the caliber required in a teacher. He lacked knowledge in certain areas.

When the older rabbi heard this he comforted the young man. "I assume you had difficulty because of the tiring journey. Why don't you rest up at your inn? Come back in a few days and I'm sure you will get the position."

The days passed but the young man did not return. Instead the rabbi went to the inn and found him. "Why haven't we seen you?" he asked.

"Thank you, rabbi," the young man said. "You have caused me to open my eyes and see things as they are. Now I know my place and I will be going home."

"Now, don't do anything precipitate," said the rabbi. "Stay in the city and you will surely get the position."

The rabbi arranged for an experienced tutor to teach the young man the area he needed to study. While he was learning, the rabbi paid all his expenses.

When the young man was tested once again, he passed

with flying colors and was offered a fine position at the school. He became so well known, in fact, that he was offered positions by other schools as well.

Ultimately the young man chose a school closer to his family. Before he left the city he came to the rabbi to thank him. In the course of their conversation he asked why the rabbi had done so much for him.

"When you first came to me and asked for my forgiveness I told you that I forgave you completely and I bore you no grudge whatsoever," replied the rabbi. "And, indeed, I said what I truly felt. But a person cannot control his feelings, and I was afraid that deep down I might still bear you something of a grudge. Now there is a saying that by taking an action one can undo one's thoughts. I therefore sought to do you a favor so as to remove any possible grudge from my heart. It is part of man's nature that if he helps another, he grows to love the one he has helped."

There were tears in the young man's eyes as he shook hands with the learned rabbi. "I, too, have learned to love. I learned by example. Your example. Thank you again."

Very often taking charge requires this very ability to learn to forgive. Forgiveness is not a simple task. While the rabbi had to forgive a public humiliation that was soon put to rights by his thunderous welcome and the esteem in which he was held in the city, most Chadults do not have the same level of acceptance to balance their hurt.

Most Chadults had their humiliating moments in the privacy of their homes as they were growing up. Some were never even given the dignity of an apology by the parent who was short-tempered or irascible. These Chadults often grow up to be much like their parents—people with long memories and short fuses.

How are they to deal appropriately—kindly and fairly—with their aging parent or parents after years of hurt? Are they capable of learning that to help another can bring about love?

Certainly, any decision that includes the component of love will be well thought out and frequently kinder than one made without love. But sometimes it takes more than love to do what is right. It takes, at times, a tough stance, the ability to see the big picture, to look into the future with the knowledge that it might become even bleaker.

In an ideal world the parent would take responsibility for his longterm care. Like the goal-oriented man who put his wishes in writing, he would tell his children exactly what he wanted and hope they would agree to do as he asked.

He would lay out a plan that was workable financially and physically for all his children. He might, if his children were truly fortunate, take a lesson from the rabbi and understand true forgiveness. He would know that there might be wounds to heal while he was still able to talk through painful issues. Although they might be of no importance to him—indeed, many aging parents are surprised when their adult children remember incidents that to the parent were trivial—he would understand that Chadults are more eager to be caregivers if the slate is cleaner than it has been.

What the rabbi accomplished was the feat of a truly disciplined man who had spent his life learning to understand how human beings behave. He had been given the privilege of the leisure to examine *himself* and learn about his personal responses.

Most Chadults do not have this privilege. We act and react and rush from place to place and from issue to issue, leaving many things unanswered and unresolved. We do not slow down to allow ourselves to grow and learn to love and alleviate the pain and hurt.

Very often our responses as Chadults are reactionary rather than thoughtful or reasonable. When we see our parents in distress and we recognize the time has come when we must get involved, we feel angry or panicked and trapped.

Families have attempted to "all meet under one roof" and see what is best for Mom or Dad. The time for telephone calls to be made as needed has ended.

Gathering in one place can work very well, but the purpose of the gathering must not be lost. Nor, in angry situations, must the parent be victimized by vitriolic statements.

Noreen was in her fifties when it came time to make some important family decisions about her father. He had lived alone for some years as a widower, but now he was ill and knew the time for living alone was past. His funds were meager and he saw almost no options that were comfortable.

Although Noreen was one of four Chadults who would all be involved, she believed her issues with her father carried the greatest pain.

The oldest child, she was born just after Norman, her father, had been shipped overseas during the Second World War. By the time he came home, she was five years old. She believed that she and Ethel, her mother, ran the little world in which they lived. She slept in her mother's bed every night. Her mother would get up in the morning and walk her to school. The two of them would decide what they would have for dinner. And so on. Ethel, although constantly talking about Daddy and how much she loved him, had treated Noreen more as a peer than a child.

Then the big moment arrived. Daddy came home from the war!

It was only to be expected that once he arrived Noreen would be sent back to her own bed, and peer decisions would now be made by the peers—Mom and Dad.

From then on, Noreen and her father competed for the attention of Ethel. Noreen felt displaced and was too young to verbalize how she was feeling. In that era it was rare to send a child—or anyone—to a social worker or psychologist.

In fact, if people did seek out such resources it was always done secretly, as if there were something shameful about it.

Norman had no idea why his daughter did not respond to him. Most of the other servicemen's children, especially the girls, were clinging to and hugging their fathers. As he saw it, he had made many overtures only to have them rejected. Finally, after a long talk with his wife, he decided the anger in his home was becoming overpowering. He would just let his little girl be. If she wanted no part of him, he would have to learn to live with that, and he stopped trying so hard with his only child. Ethel was unhappy because he was so hurt, so she, too, withdrew from Noreen. Then, in quick succession, three more children were born.

The younger children knew nothing of the problems between Noreen and their parents. They only knew they were brought into a warm and loving home that contained a lot of laughter. Why Noreen sat off to one side was a mystery in which they did not wish to become involved.

The outcome? There was a family of five. Plus Noreen.

Outwardly she acted as if she didn't mind her isolation. But inwardly the pain was tearing her apart.

When she was old enough she left the area and moved to New York, where she became a highly regarded freelance writer. She seemed able to get inside the people she interviewed and understand their pain.

Noreen spent very little time thinking about her family back home. Certainly she was invited to confirmations and weddings, but only occasionally did she accept. She did not know her nieces and nephews well enough for their milestones to matter to her. She was too envious of her siblings.

She would occasionally drop short notes to her mother. These were always courteous and formal. After all, she felt that her mother had taken sides, picking the father instead of Noreen. And Noreen couldn't let that go.

But in more recent times people have learned to address painful issues and feelings more openly. It is common now to seek some mental health guidance. It was when she sought such help that Noreen learned why she was in such pain.

Like the rabbi, she came to believe that she had to take an action or there could be no undoing her negative thoughts.

So she decided to visit her family in order to talk with her father. She had to let him know that as a child she had not understood that he was only assuming his rightful place in the family. No one had prepared her for this change in her life. Her mother, now dead, had just assumed they would return to a normal family structure. She had not explained to Noreen that they had fallen into an unusual and temporary circumstance.

Noreen arrived to find the entire family in an uproar. Since she had very little contact with them she did not know her father's health was slowly deteriorating from Parkinson's disease. None of her siblings was able to care for him because each of them had a demanding full-time job.

What was to be done? The siblings were all sitting in their father's living room attempting to have a family meeting when Noreen walked in. She had not called or written to say that she was coming because she did not want them to pick her up at the airport. She, in fact, wanted nothing from them. She had come only to talk with her father.

There was silence in the room as she entered and dropped her suitcases on the floor. She looked from her siblings to their spouses and then to Norman. All their faces were blank with amazement.

"Why, what's the problem here?" she asked. "Did I interrupt a family party? If you ask me, it looks more like a family wake!"

"Oh, shut up!" said Wally, her oldest brother. "We're in the middle of a family meeting. We've got a crisis on our hands and we need a solution."

Noreen's years of writing about people and her years of therapy suddenly kicked in. She looked from one to the other and realized that yes, indeed, there was a problem. Furthermore, when she looked at her father and saw the trembling in his hands and the fear in his eyes, she understood at once that the issue revolved around him.

"Can I be part of the discussion, or would you rather I leave? I'll understand either way," she said quietly.

"No," said her father. "I want you to stay."

Noreen was shocked at his slurred speech and the lack of timbre in his voice.

"How about the rest of you? Do you want me to stay?"

Sisters and brothers looked at their spouses. Then, one by one, they nodded. After all, even though she had distanced herself, Noreen was still family.

Noreen pulled in a chair from the dining room and sat down. "Now, what is the problem here? Can I help?"

Janet, the sister closer in age to her, said simply, "The problem is that Dad has Parkinson's and can't be left alone any longer. He needs help with his meals. He needs someone to stay overnight because he is afraid. He needs to be someplace where he has company so he can talk to people instead of being alone in this house all day. He can't get out anymore. That's the problem, Noreen."

"Is that what you see, Dad? Is that the problem?"

"Well, I see it all a little differently," he said in his low, slow voice. "Sure, I need some help, but I don't want to go anywhere. I don't want to live with anyone. I want to manage on my own."

"But, Dad, that's impossible," said Wally. "You're spilling food everywhere. You know that."

Noreen said very little as all the others spoke. They were quite emotional. She felt like an interloper, but she did have some useful suggestions she wished to make.

When her siblings were finally quiet, she asked if there were any good day-care facilities in the area. She was told there were, but how would their father get there? Who would help him dress in the morning? Who would be there for him at the end of the day?

"Well, Dad doesn't seem immobilized to me," she said. "Dad, are you able to do anything for yourself?"

"If you call walking and talking doing for myself, I can certainly do that! These people are making a big fuss about nothing!"

"It looks like *something* to me," she said gently. "I wonder if there is a high school senior who lives around here and drives. I wonder if he could come before school and give Dad whatever help he needs. Maybe he or someone else could come back after school and help with dinner and getting Dad ready for bed. Dad seems like he can manage on his own after that."

"Well, that's what I've been trying to tell them. You came at just the right minute. They wanted to send me to a nursing home. I'm not ready for that yet!" Norman agreed to the student idea, providing the person was a male. He said he didn't want young girls fussing over him.

Of course this solution raised many areas of concern: how to find the right day-care center, how to make certain the young helpers were reliable, what to do if Dad needed help during the night. All of these issues had to addressed. But Noreen had opened a window to let her family see the options.

They got busy the next day and found a fine day-care center that provided lunch and cots for napping and had a full range of activities for people with various disabilities. It was a point of honor with this center that no one sat idly watching others working on pleasurable projects.

The family called the high school guidance counselor and the teacher supervising students who needed jobs. To their pleasant surprise they had fifteen young men to interview by the end of the week and of that group felt comfortable with at least seven.

Their father was very pleased. He was not yet ready for an "all-night baby-sitter." He wanted to be in his own home, alone, as long as he was able.

The family was effusive in its thanks to their oldest sister. Janet summed it up best: "I guess since we all see one another every day we simply got stuck repeating the same old things. You gave us some new information and a new approach. Besides, you were the only one who really listened to Dad about his wishes. Thanks. I'd love it if you would stay a while instead of doing one of your usual flying visits."

Noreen smiled. "I planned to stay for ten days or so. I want to be with Dad."

Her family was taken aback by this. On her rare visits she stayed in a hotel. Now here she was wanting to stay with the person she liked the least.

Noreen saw their bewilderment. "I really have some things to talk over with him. I'd like to do it slowly. Don't worry, I won't upset him. At least, I hope I won't."

Janet reached forward and touched her arm. "Somehow I trust you. I don't think you'll make his condition worse."

Because they had time, Noreen did not have to yell at her father about feeling pushed away. She talked to him adult to adult. She certainly let him know what had happened and how hurt she felt. But the years, in her case, had been kind, and the sting had gone out of her pain. She was able to tell him how *she* perceived her childhood and how *she* felt abandoned when he returned from the service.

Her father was not a fool and he listened to her over those ten days. He did not attempt to interrupt her with defenses of his and his wife's behavior . . . especially in the beginning.

When he felt she had gotten the poison out of her system he took her hand across the kitchen table. "I loved your mother very much and she loved me. I guess she was not very wise. She was so young when I went overseas that she probably did not even think about you as a small person with feelings. You were her companion, and when I returned *I* was her companion. She probably just assumed you would return to being her child. But hearing you tell it, I guess it just wasn't that simple for you. I'm truly sorry, Noreen. I imagine that's why you've stayed away. Hell, I'd probably have done the same thing. I only hope you'll be part of this family now that we've talked."

Noreen had tears in her eyes as she nodded. "I don't know why I waited so long. I wish I could have explained this to Mom."

"Honey, there's a time for everything, and you can't rush anything before its time. Just remember that—and pour me a cup of coffee."

Noreen smiled and gave her father the first unsolicited hug they had ever shared.

While she had endured many years of pain, Noreen in the end had the wonderful luxury of time. Time to sort through her feelings. Time to receive appropriate therapy. Time to gain wisdom. And, most important, time to express her feelings to a man who had the time to listen.

Often when Chadults arrange a family meeting it is very tense. Unknowingly, Noreen walked into just such a poignant moment in her own family. In the worst situations things are said and done that might have been better left unsaid and undone. While the parent may have been a larger-than-life bully to his children, there have been many situations when family meetings turn into unproductive "Let's get even with Dad" sessions.

One Chadult will suddenly have a painful memory flash through her mind; rather than leaving it for another time, she will verbalize it.

Often, this starts a chain of responses. Unfortunately, the parent is rarely defended because each child is busy recalling his or her own hurts and pains.

In such a situation there is a gray-haired person who was either a good parent or a bad parent—or possibly a parent who is judged by the child and the child's emotions rather than by the facts. The parent is now at the mercy of this group of people who, ostensibly having come to discuss positive alternatives, end up excoriating the aging mother or father for things that cannot be undone. And nothing positive is accomplished.

If all the siblings had a rocky upbringing it might be wise for each Chadult to meet with the parent separately first so Mom doesn't feel ganged up on. At this private meeting the Chadult can discuss in a moderate manner what was so hurtful.

If he can begin with the statement "There is really nothing

you can do about any of this now, but I have to get it off my chest so we can go forward in a better way," and then *calmly* discuss what the recollection is, he may make progress and sometimes even reach closure.

But painful memories should be dealt with in a private meeting, not one that is threatening. When you have this conversation, remember you are facing your parent's entire future, not some little block in time. Remember, too, that the future holds only moderately things that are positive and exciting. It is a downhill run, and we can only hope that the slopes will be gentle.

You must decide when to visit with your parent privately. Some Chadults claim it is better to meet before the family conference. Others think that talking afterward has the best results.

One social worker describes a family meeting for a now wheelchair-bound mother that sounded like the legal time to hunt deer. It was open season on Mother!

Rhonda's three daughters had spoken together almost daily for more than a month about the problem, but none of these small conversations had included their mother. The older woman, now frail and sick, was about to feel the full force of her children's unhappiness with their upbringing when they decided to confront her together.

Just as human beings eat one bite at a time, so it is often necessary to discuss challenging problems in the same way. Cramming an entire slice of bread into your mouth, then attempting to chew it, is ludicrous. So is trying to tell a parent in one dose what has been decided about her future.

As the three sisters drove to their mother's apartment they continued their what-to-do-about-Mother conversation. When they got there, they let themselves in—each sister had a key— and found Mother watching television.

Andrea, the oldest, walked over to the set and snapped it off without asking for permission.

"We've got to talk, Mom. We need to decide what to do about your problem," she said.

"What problem is that?" asked her mother.

"You know what we're talking about," snapped Justine. "It's got to be obvious we can't keep this up any longer."

"Mom, we can't keep running back and forth the way we've been doing. It's just too hard," said Shelly.

Their mother, although physically impaired, was still a bright and knowing woman. She looked from one to another and said, "I raised all of you. There was room in *my* house for all of you. Isn't it strange how one mother can care for three kids and three kids can't care for one woman? It's like some inverted arithmetic problem, isn't it?"

The sisters looked at one another. No one knew quite how to respond. If adult women could squirm like little children they assuredly were squirming.

Finally, Andrea could stand it no longer. Her discomfort cut the filter between her mind and her mouth. "Sure, there was always room! Room for you to criticize me and make fun of my weight in front of my friends. Room to always take Justine's part in an argument and not mine. Oh, yeah, there was lots of room!"

Andrea's face was red with anger as she spoke her unguarded words. Her mother had turned ashen.

"Well, she may have sided with me, but she never let me forget for a moment that I was stupid and you were the smart one. No matter what grades I brought home they always could have been better. Isn't that the truth, Mother?"

Their mother could feel the trembling in her hands become more intense. They were all so angry. What was going on here?

Shelly looked from one to the other. "Oh, you poor dears. Life was so terrible for you. I'm ten years younger than Justine. By the time I came on the scene our parents' marriage only had a year left, and I was raised without my father! You were all too busy for me then. When I came to my mother with a problem she said, 'Go away, I have too much on my mind right now.' I don't feel sorry for you two at all! Or for you, Mother, for that matter!"

Rhonda began to cry. "Why are you here? What do you want?"

But her daughters were far from through venting the years of anger they had never expressed. Every unresolved issue was hurled at the mother. The sisters were tripping over one another to make their points.

Rhonda could feel herself becoming more and more ill. Her emphysema was making breathing even more difficult because of the stress she was experiencing. She grew disoriented and it became harder to answer as words were shot at her by her daughters, who did not pause for breath between indictments.

Finally, she could take it no longer. "I don't know why you came," she said in a reedy voice. "But I know you have to leave. Maybe you can come another day when we can talk. I have to go to bed."

Instead of asking for their help she turned her chair and rolled it into her bedroom, slamming the door behind her. She pushed the chair as close to the bed as possible and with Herculean effort rolled onto it from the wheelchair. She did not bother to get out of her clothing. She just needed to get away from all that animosity and lie down quietly.

Her daughters were startled back to the present when the door slammed. They looked at each other, shamefaced. "Now what the hell did I do?" Andrea said angrily.

"You shot off your big mouth," Justine responded.

"No, we all did," said Shelly, the youngest and the peacemaker.

"I'm going in there to say I'm sorry and kiss her good night. I'll tell her we'll talk another day," she added.

When Shelly went into the bedroom she found her mother just lying there looking pale and ill. She apologized and left when Rhonda said she needed nothing from her at that time.

The next morning the mother telephoned the local lung association. She asked for help in finding a decent nursing home. Explaining that she was wheelchair-bound, she also asked if a volunteer would come and take her to visit some of the homes in her area. She was fortunate; a woman came to help her. They searched over a span of several weeks. Ultimately, Rhonda decided on a clean home that seemed well run. She signed all the admission papers.

When she got home she rested and then called her daughters and said they needed to come and talk. When they arrived each apologized for her raging.

"That's not necessary. How you picture your childhood is how it must have been for you. I can't change that. But I *can* change the responsibility for taking care of me. It is just not fair, after what I heard from you. I am going to a nursing home. I have signed the papers. I am moving in two days. I hope you will come and visit."

The sisters were dumbfounded. They were convinced their mother was just having a tantrum and would change her mind. But she did not. The move to the nursing home came about just as she planned. Ultimately the sisters did come to visit. At first they did so with guilt, but after a while they saw that Rhonda had indeed made a good decision. They were now free to live their own lives and free to visit comfortably, knowing all their mother's needs were being met.

Family meetings should never turn into such shouting matches and such moments of negative triumph. A family meeting requires grace and caring and everyone's acknowledgment that the parent's interest is the primary concern.

Family members should not simply show up one night. Instead it would be kinder to call and let Mom or Dad know that you feel it is necessary to get together and talk about how things need to be handled since he or she is so unwell.

Don't turn the telephone call into a threat. Speak gently and yet firmly to let Mom know this subject can no longer be ignored. It is time to make some decisions. You will want the meeting to be a productive one.

- Be prepared. Come to the meeting with some carefully thought out ideas of your own. Ask friends and members of organizations to which you belong about alternatives they may have chosen or heard about.
- The question of money can never be ignored; it might be wise to make an appointment with a financial planner, who can help stretch tight dollars to their maximum.
- Leave your grudges and angers at home. Also, do not allow your parent to bait you and push guilt upon you. If you know your agenda is pure and does not include spite or revenge you will feel more comfortable. If, however, you do feel these things, see a counselor before the meeting. Many are available at little or no cost.
- If you fear there will be angry feelings expressed, ask a hospital social worker or a private counselor to sit

in as an adviser. Often when a stranger is present, whether professionally trained or not, family members remember their manners just a trifle better.

- Unless some family member has an objection, bring a tape recorder or video camera to the meeting. There can be no "he said, she said" afterward, because you have it on tape. This can also help Mom or Dad remember how decisions were made.

- Set a time limit on the meeting. You cannot decide everything in one session, nor should you try to. You are, after all, dealing with the rest of someone's life.

- Make certain there are no interruptions. Turn on the answering machine or take the phone off the hook during the meeting. Don't allow distractions.

- Explain to Mom or Dad why you feel some further help is needed. Don't do this as an accusation. State the facts kindly and matter-of-factly. If the issue is whether Mom is eating appropriately, let her know you are *concerned*. This is not a matter of her being at fault. You are worried. That attitude can make all the difference in how you are heard.

The Commandments tell us to honor our father and mother. Sadly, it is not always possible to love them. Circumstances may have arisen that made it appropriate for you to distance yourself from them. But you can always honor them for the fact that they brought *you* into being. They gave you life.

Allow that fact to hang like a soft white cloud over the entire meeting. It will gentle all of you and help you to use clarity when it is time to make decisions.

Chapter 5

STAGES

—◆—

*There is an hour in each man's
life appointed to make his happiness,
if then he seize it.*
—Beaumont and Fletcher

What is a crisis to one person may be laughable to the next. How often have we seen well-dressed men and women step into their expensive cars looking distraught because they were going to be late for a luncheon?

Late for a luncheon? Now, that's not a very good thing, you might think. But then you walk farther down the road and you see a homeless woman pushing her shopping cart. What would she make of being late for a luncheon? you might wonder.

Still farther down the road you pass a funeral procession proceding in a slow, stately manner. You smile as the expensively dressed man in his expensive car looks impatiently at his watch and has to wait until the procession has passed him by!

So few people are able to seize the moment. So few are able to understand that now is all we have. Yesterday is history and tomorrow is mystery!

While the lessons of history are always our primers, we cannot invariably continue to say, "But we always did it this way," or "We always felt that way." Life is fluid. Things do not stay the same. Life is about change and relationships and aging. History is that part of us that we can look back on when we are happy or sad or merely in a reminiscing mood.

Reminiscing can leave us strong or vulnerable.

If we remember things that brought us pleasure and we feel good, the trip into our memory is obviously positive. But what if it leaves us feeling vulnerable? What if it leaves us comparing what was with what is? What if we remembered ourselves young and running, but now have to look down at our walker or wheelchair? The pain of such a memory can drain us of our vitality and sometimes our wish to live.

In order for Chadults to understand fully what their parents are experiencing as they age and become infirm, it is necessary to look at the stages they and their parents are going through.

In many instances these stages are no different than those so frequently mentioned in discussions about death and dying. It is important to remember a story Elisabeth Kübler-Ross, who wrote the classic *On Death and Dying*, tells. After giving much thought to how she was going to write her great book, she decided to begin with denial, since so often people say, "Oh no, this is not really happening to me or to the person I love!"

As she wrote her book Kübler-Ross tried to follow the stages of grief, focusing each chapter on the prevalent emotion of each stage. She covered anger and guilt and depression and acceptance.

When the book hit the stores like dynamite she was inundated with mail. People wrote to thank her, to share their own personal stories with her, or just to feel connected to this great woman.

But what astounded Kübler-Ross was the number of letters from people who felt panicked because they were not experiencing the emotions in the sequence in which she had written about them. People were horrified if they felt guilt before denial! What was wrong with them? How come they were so out of the ordinary?

Dr. Kübler-Ross actually wrote a second book, *Questions and Answers on Death and Dying*, to clear up this issue.

People are human. We are not robots programmed to feel a certain emotion at nine A.M. and then another at eleven. We feel what we feel because of the mix of circumstances around us. We feel what we feel because of the weather. We feel what we feel if our friends have been considerate. We feel what we feel if our family has been loving. Sometimes we feel what we feel because we are the people we are. In other words, we react. We act. We live through a wide range of emotions daily as long as we are alert and alive.

Interestingly, according to many gerontology experts, the emotions we experience as Chadults are no different than what we experience over a death. We are watching someone we love, or at least knew in a different context, begin the inevitable process of aging.

With aging comes change. Since most of us are creatures of habit we become used to the familiar. Aging attacks our senses on several levels. We see the process as it slowly creeps up on someone we love, and the deterioration can be painful. We know the inevitable outcome of aging is death.

Our society is so fraught with rushing and running and trying to get everything done that sometimes we are absolutely shocked to see that Mother has changed so radically in "so short a time." Actually, Mother has been changing slowly for some time, but we are so busy that we do not even notice the changes. After all, she has not taken any major falls. She is still driving and preparing her own meals.

We barely notice that she seems to be calling us a bit more frequently. We don't look for subtle signs of change like spots on her clothing that at one time never would have been there.

Lois, a wealthy, designer-clad woman, was a member of a country club. She played cards there several times a week and rarely lost a canasta tournament. Her mind was sharp and clear and her friends marveled that her play had not slowed down at all despite her being seventy years old.

What they were not seeing, however, was a more subtle change. While Lois still went to the hairdresser weekly, and therefore still looked good on the surface, no one noticed that her clothing was becoming spotted. Since she was a widow there was no one to point out that such and such a dress needed to be cleaned.

Lois had one child, a daughter, Stacie, who lived out of state. While the two tried to maintain a relationship and visit frequently, their busy schedules did not allow them to see each other as much as they might have wished.

Lois's daughter, who would fly in and fly out in a matter of days, either never attached importance or simply did not notice that her mother had begun to be inattentive to her clothing. Their time together was so limited that often they just stayed in their robes in Lois's home and talked from morning to night.

Stacie, while sorry to be away, had the comfortable feeling that her mother was doing well. She was fully occupied and her telephone rang fairly frequently.

"I would feel worse about being so far away if I didn't know how many people cared about her," said Stacie. "As long as she is active I don't worry overly about her deterioration."

Stacie, of course, was correct to some degree, but signs of change that are quite subtle need watching, and Lois's seeming disregard for the appearance of her clothing was one such sign.

She would show up at the finest parties, brain alert, hair done, makeup nicely applied—but on her garments were spots that were obviously not new.

One longtime friend, Irene, happened to notice a large stain on Lois's dress and knew it had been there for several weeks. She herself had accidentally spilled some coffee in that same spot. Since they were good friends, Irene went up to Lois and jokingly asked if she needed money to pay her dry-cleaning bill. She, Irene, would gladly pay for the cleaning if only Lois would get the spot out. "Haven't you heard of Lady Macbeth and 'Out, damned spot'?" she joked.

Lois looked at her, bewildered. "I don't wear clothes with spots on them and you know it, Irene. My things are always being sent to the cleaner."

Irene was taken aback by the fervent tone in Lois's voice.

Had she but realized it, the tone was defensive. Lois had not studied her wardrobe as her maid had always done. Now that she was a widow she was anxious about finances, and had dismissed the maid. There was nothing wrong with Lois's eyes. She had merely stopped paying attention.

Lack of attention to detail can be an early warning sign of aging. It is one of the easier ones for a Chadult to handle. In a case such as this one, a Chadult can help the parent develop a rigid schedule for when clothing is checked and sent to the cleaner. Once the pattern is set we can do away with the Lady Macbeth syndrome.

How often have we heard that "clothes make the man"? Some years back there was a fashion called the Nehru jacket. Unlike a regular jacket with lapels, it had a high collar that rested on the neck. Most men who liked high fashion owned at least one of these.

But like all trends, this one also saw its time come and go. Twenty years after the trend had seen its demise, Dave, now a man in his sixties, was still wearing the same beige Nehru jacket. What looked attractive when he was forty-five lost its luster when it faded both from style and from wear. Dave looked like an old man fighting to recapture his lost youth—and no one would tell him. He was divorced. His children lived in different cities. How was he to know?

One weekend his daughter, Elyse, and her children came to visit from out of town and as a surprise they brought along some home movies that were taken at her wedding. Dave was delighted to see the movies. Some of his friends had since died and he wanted to enjoy seeing them dancing and having a good time once again.

Elyse prepared dinner and all of them, including his three grandchildren aged ten, twelve, and fourteen, sat down to watch the wedding movie. As soon as the pictures of the Nehru jackets came on Dave's grandchildren doubled up with laughter. "Grandpa, you look like you're in a time warp!" said the oldest boy, who loved him dearly. "You're still wearing the same jacket they're wearing in the movie! We've got to get you with it!"

The other two youngsters simply laughed and laughed.

Dave's daughter could see that her father's feelings had been hurt and she took his hand. "I didn't know how to tell you. I didn't want to make you feel bad. But you are a pack rat, and if something isn't torn you keep wearing it until it's ragged. Dad, we've got to get you 'with it.' "

This was a revelation to Dave. He hadn't even noticed that times had gone by and styles had changed. He only knew he was comfortable in his well-broken-in jacket.

There is nothing wrong with being comfortable. After all, that is one of the goals each of us strives to accomplish. But still we must encourage our parents to look around and see what is current and how they are reflecting these new trends in their own lives.

How much judging and encouraging is enough when Chadults view their parents? One man who is well into his eighties likes nothing better than to wear tight blue jeans and all manner of Western silver-and-turquoise jewelry. His white hair is long and he ties it in a ponytail. Now, this would indeed be high fashion and admirable if he lived in New Mexico or Arizona. But he doesn't. He lives in New York. He attends the symphony in this garb. He goes to fashionable gatherings dressed the same way.

While he is welcomed and accepted outwardly—he is a major donor to many charities—people shake their heads after he leaves. He has crossed the age line. People think it is time for him to give up that cool look and dress like a conservative gentleman. But no one dares tell him so.

Perhaps he is better off going about his business just as he is, for he seems content. Yet is that the appropriate look for an eighty-something man?

He has grown children, a son and a daughter, both married. Both couples are part of the society scene also. They confess to shuddering when they see him trying to look like "a young stud," as the son put it.

"We go places and there he is dressed in that phony Western getup. I mean, in black-tie places. I guess his money makes it acceptable. If he looked like that and was a street person, people would look at him as if he were a freak!"

There are people who would disagree with these Chadults. They might say, "As long as the man is still interested in the world around him and is still willing to go to social functions, why is his attire such a big deal?"

Others might think or say, "What is the purpose of dressing like a man forty years younger than his true age?" They might wonder if he is in denial about aging.

If people like his Chadult children were to explore the concept with him, he might ask them, "What is wrong with looking young? We live in a youth-oriented society. I'm just staying in line with how people think and feel! Youth feels good and safe. Maybe I like that, too." It's hard to argue with this. Yet somewhere there must be room for a balance. Should Chadults be their parent's keepers?

There is a older woman, named Alice, who goes regularly to the beauty shop, where she has her hair tinted and streaked. She dresses in tight jeans and enticing sweaters. Her face is so lined that no makeup can cover it. But that is not her problem. Her hairdresser and other shop clients can smell her as soon as she walks through the door. She is loaded with perfume. Expensive perfume. But even that is not enough to cover her body odor.

She refuses to bathe.

She has had numerous attendants. All have been fired by her daughter, Rita, because they have been unable to make her take a shower, sponge bath, or tub bath. The mother and daughter have had screaming matches about this problem. But the mother prevails. "I'm just fine the way I am. I wear my Chanel and no one can tell. I don't like the feel of water against my skin! That's why I never use the pool or go into the ocean when we vacation!"

Rita throws up her hands and once again feels she is losing this battle. She has long given up reminding her mother how fastidiously clean she had always kept her house and her children. Rita can remember the times she was sent back to her room to change her dress because there was a spot on it.

They had had many arguments in the daughter's formative years about what the daughter considered excessive tidiness.

Not only was her daughter expected to take a bath nightly, she was expected to take a shower afterward to rinse off the "nasty" bathwater.

Her mother demanded no more of the daughter than she did of herself. She practiced the same bathing routine. That is why the daughter is so shocked at this change.

The parents were divorced when Rita was quite young. Alice was a strong-minded, independent woman who had built a thriving clothing business. The idea of trying to "control" her mother was somewhat intimidating to Rita because of the years during which she had been unable to do so.

"It feels like a teenaged rebellion to me," she says, and perhaps in a way that is indeed the case.

This question of bathing seems to affect any number of older people. Some are in Assisted Living apartments. Amanda, one such woman, lives in luxurious surroundings and refuses to bathe. Her daughter-in-law, Judith, came to visit one day after being away for several weeks, and was outraged. Judith reeked and her apartment reeked. When she went to the manager he threw his hands up and said there was nothing he could do.

"We try to coax her," he said. "People refuse to sit with her in the dining room. Nothing seems to make a difference. She says she's afraid of falling when she gets out of the tub. She says she's afraid of water touching her skin. Was she always like this?"

"Not so far as I've heard," Judith replied. "In fact, she was a cleanliness freak if anything."

The two of them decided Amanda needed an assistant to help her bathe. But then Judith got a call from the manager telling her the plan simply was not working. Amanda would not get in the tub and she would not get out of the tub. At least four different assistants who were trained to give baths had given up.

The daughter-in-law finally hit on a solution. She got Gilbert, her husband, involved. "She's your mother," she pointed out. "I want you to go and be tough. She might listen to you."

When Amanda's son went to see her—and it had been a while—he was shocked by the odor. He began to scream at his mother. He had planned to speak rationally and give her all the health reasons for bathing, but this plan went down the drain when he walked through the door. The smell was fierce—rotten eggs, decaying flesh. No wonder the manager had ended the conversation with his wife with a threat of eviction.

The son verbally lambasted his mother to the point where she began to cry, and he kept right on going. Finally, Amanda agreed to have an attendant come right up and give her a tub bath. She had tried to negotiate for a sponge bath. But he would not hear of it. That wouldn't even come close to taking away the smell.

He sat in the living room as the two women worked in the bathroom. He could hear his mother crying and the other woman coaxing. They stayed there for half an hour. When his mother finally emerged wearing a clean white terrycloth robe he went up to her and kissed her. "Mom, I'm sorry I got so angry. I couldn't even get near enough to you to kiss. Now let's get out of this apartment and have someone come in and clean it so we are rid of the smell."

Amanda agreed. From that time on Gilbert made it a point to visit twice a week, and Amanda knew each visit meant taking a bath and having her apartment cleaned. In the end, mother and son found time to visit on a friendly level and her later years proved warmer than she had imagined because of this relationship.

There are problems that arise, however, that have not yet been solved. Nursing homes have very strict guidelines on how residents must be treated. It is generally impossible to forcibly bathe a resident who resists being cleaned. Resident's rights always prevail. If the state or federal government were to ask this resident how she was being treated and she told them she was being forced to do anything, the nursing facility would be investigated and possibly fined. These issues are of great concern to nursing home employees and families of residents as well.

Frequently social workers will try to intervene, as will doctors and nurses. But some people, like Amanda, will simply insist on their way. Many people in nursing homes do not have the kind of involved relatives who will come as the son did to battle his mother until she listened to him. Instead, it is up to the professional staff to coax and cajole. The rules are so strict they can do no more than that.

In general, when Chadults are in denial about their parents' aging it is because it is frightening to see a loss of function. Chadults often have unreasonable expectations and want things to remain as they always were. But if we can understand that change is inevitable, perhaps we will not make so many excuses not to visit our parents because "seeing them getting old is so painful."

Another important change that occurs is the sense of loss we feel when our parents no longer act the way we always knew them to act. If they were volatile, we see that as the norm. If they were quiet and peace-loving people, we see that as the norm. Even if they were erratic, we learned long ago to live with that kind of behavior.

As parents get older new behaviors arise. They are frightening because they are not familiar. We often become angry and think to ourselves, "She's just doing that to make me mad." Or, "She really could remember if she tried. It's just a game." Or even, "She's just trying to get my attention."

In other words, it's easy for a Chadult to think that the older person is deliberately doing something to him. Certainly many people become manipulative as they age. Many seniors will tell you it is a survival technique! But rather than having a positive outcome, this behavior, whether intentional or not, brings out the worst in Chadults.

Rosalyn went to visit Lucille, her mother, one afternoon. This was not something she loved doing, but she felt it was her duty. She had her own key and used it. When she walked through the door she saw her mother sitting in front of the television eating a bowl of soup. No sooner did the mother look up and see her daughter than she took a mouthful of soup and spat it at her. Rosalyn was furious.

The family had hired a woman who came in daily at mealtime. She was nowhere to be found that afternoon, but her telephone number was on the refrigerator. Rosalyn called, and the woman said she had quit. "She spits her food at me all the time and there are nice, well-mannered people who need my help. I will not be spat on like that!"

Rosalyn turned to Lucille. "Do you realize what you've done? You're spitting like a little girl. Melinda just told me you did that to her and she quit. Now what are we going to do?"

Lucille looked at her with a somewhat blank stare.

"But I don't like the soup," she said.

"What difference does that make? You don't spit food. You know better!"

And there may very well lie the fallacy. At one time Mother *did* know better. But does she know better now? Without a thorough examination there is no way to answer that question. The problem lies with the built-in mind-set of the Chadult. Mom is just "acting" that way and she could change if she wanted to.

This always brings to mind the "Serenity Prayer," in which we ask to know the difference between what we can and cannot change. If we would get that straight in our minds perhaps we could let go of the process of pounding brick walls and trying to alter what cannot be changed. We can learn despite our resistance, despite our efforts, despite our wishes, that Mom or Dad is in a different mental or physical place. We may not like it, but that is the *new* reality.

Gloria, who was in her nineties, fell and banged her head. After the fall she needed a walker to help her keep her balance, but mentally she seemed fine—until suddenly, two weeks later, she could not communicate. She was hallucinating and thrashing so violently that she needed to be hospitalized and restrained.

Denise was the only one of her children who lived in the same city, and the years of caring for and worrying about her mother had worn her out. She was short-tempered and impatient and frustrated with her mother's stubbornness. While this same tenacity may have helped Gloria reach the age of ninety, it became increasingly difficult to interact with her as a concerned Chadult.

Over a period of a quarter century Gloria took what once had been habits, like being careful about money, to the extreme, because now she even hoarded food despite having ample funds in the bank.

Because Denise was unwilling to attribute this sudden change to the fall, she called in a new gerontologist who examined Gloria thoroughly. He, like Denise, was not convinced the erratic behavior resulted from the fall. He asked the daughter to check on what her mother had been eating.

"I was in shock," Denise recalls. "Her refrigerator was stocked with leftovers that were weeks old. Food from when we took her to brunch or dinner. I couldn't even tell what some of the things were! We believe it was some kind of food poisoning that triggered her system to respond that way."

Since Gloria was in the hospital she had no access to spoiled food; in a matter of five days or so her mind was clear and she could not understand what had happened.

"She keeps insisting it was from the fall and I'm tired of arguing with her," her daughter says. "We'll just have to make sure she doesn't take doggie bags from restaurants again!"

Without the proper examination and the tests that were given there is no telling what diagnosis would have been rendered. Doctors might even have agreed with Gloria that her problems were a result of the fall.

"What makes me angriest of all," Denise says, "is that I get this feeling inside that my mother is doing something to get even with me. I can never visit her enough or do enough or be enough. That's just the way it is. I kept thinking she was tricking me or trying to put something over on me. Now I feel foolish, but I can't swear I would believe her immediately the next time something happened.

"I just feel my mother is trying to do something to *me*. It doesn't make sense. I know that. But I don't have enough years left to live to resolve it in therapy!"

There is a story about a man who as a youngster went to a tough school. He would describe it to his children: "When I was in the sixth grade they made me count up to ten . . . by memory!"

As a story it brings a chuckle. But what if this chore is now simply too much for the parent of a Chadult? Would the Chadult believe it, or become angry at the parent's inability to complete what should be a simple task?

Vickie would reluctantly visit her mother, Arlene, at the nursing home and sit with her during her occupational therapy. No matter how much patient coaxing the staffer used, Arlene simply could not put the three thick pegs into the three round holes. Vickie would even try to help. She would hand her mother the pegs and tell her where to put them. The staffer would then try to do the same. It was all to no avail.

Finally Vickie would get so infuriated and frustrated that she would leave in a huff. "I just can't take this," she would tell the staffer. "I keep feeling that if I weren't here she would do it!" In spite of being told repeatedly that this was not the case, Vickie simply could not accept the fact that her mother had regressed so far. She felt great anger, and like other Chadults believed that her mother was doing something "to her," to spite her somehow.

Social workers and gerontologists have repeatedly stated that this type of erroneous thinking is not only agitating to the senior, it causes pain to the Chadult and makes him or her more and more reluctant to visit, especially when the parent is in a nursing home.

The lesson here is that no one is deliberately doing anything to the Chadult, and somehow this lesson must be driven home. Even if we visit someone with advanced Alzheimer's we must try to make it a loving visit so that we, the Chadults, can come away feeling loving within ourselves. If we cannot learn to do this we end up with anger and denial and a bitterness that will follow our parents, and ultimately ourselves, to the grave.

Another major area of contention between seniors and Chadults is the almost inevitable guilt that lies between them. Often parents feel that if they had their lives to live over again they would do many things differently in the upbringing of their children. Chadults often wish their parents had been stronger or weaker during their own formative years.

There is a story about two paupers who wandered from town to town begging for food and money. One was a giant of a man who had never been sick a day in his life. The other walked with a twisted foot and a hacking cough. He had never known anything but illness throughout his entire life. The giant laughed constantly at the slight, ill man, who could do nothing about his condition or the mockery he was forced to endure.

Their travels had lasted for some time when they finally reached the capital city. They arrived just when a great misfortune had befallen the king. Both his personal bodyguard and his physician had suddenly died. The king sent couriers throughout the land to gather all the strong men and physicians who might wish to compete for the vacant posts.

Out of the thousands who came forth the king finally chose a Herculean man and a physician who came with hundreds of testimonial letters. Now the king wanted to be certain he had made good choices.

The strong man suggested that the toughest and biggest man in the city be brought before him: "I will kill him with one blow from my fist."

The physician, anxious to prove his merit, said, "Give me the most helpless disabled person, and I will make him well in one week's time."

The king listened to his new appointees and sent messengers scurrying throughout the city looking for the strongest man and the most disabled person. As it turned out they found the two paupers newly arrived in the city. Both men were brought before the king, who nodded at the strong man he had appointed his new bodyguard. With one blow from his fist the bodyguard killed the giant, and after one week of excellent medical treatment the ailing man was made well again.

The moral of this story? The strength of the strong proves sometimes their misfortune, just as the weakness of the weak often brings them good fortune.

This can be very true when Chadults deal with aging parents.

Monica, who fought constantly with her mother throughout her growing-up years, found that things were no different when her mother got older. Gertrude was a tough lady and each issue that arose became a new battle.

"I know I should feel sorry for her," says Monica. "She is old. But I just don't feel kind and good and it makes me feel so guilty that I don't."

One day, however, her mother fell and had to be rushed to the hospital. Monica was notified and came quickly. Gertrude was in the emergency room, lying on a gurney, completely wrapped in a blanket and sheet.

"When I saw her my heart lurched," Monica remembers. "She looked so small and frail lying there. Could this have been the same tough cookie I had been battling with all my life? I reached over and took her hand and kissed her forehead and just kept brushing her hair off her face. I felt so tender toward her that it made me cry. What was wonderful was she was alert and knew what I was doing. She took my hand and squeezed it. Tears trickled down her cheeks too. At the moment of her weakness we came together."

Monica is very grateful for that moment, because she realized then that her mother was really aging and could die at any time. "That episode allowed me to do things that were loving and kind from then on, and I made it a point to do them. It served two purposes. I made her happy, and I made certain there would be very little guilt after she died. Catching her at such a weak time allowed us both to learn the strength of our caring."

As most mental health experts will tell you, this is not the ideal way to learn kindness and caring. It is more helpful to build a solid base of many years of caring for one another. When that base is there, doing the right thing becomes natural.

Generally that loving base is built by the parent. But dysfunctional families do exist in great numbers, and some experts feel all families have some degree of dysfunction. On the other hand, plenty of Chadults would take an oath that theirs was the perfect childhood.

The outcome of all this love parents give to their children is the kindness the parents are shown. The irony, of course, is that many parents who gave little or nothing emotionally to their children are shown as much kindness as loving parents are shown.

One action may arise from love and the other from guilt,

but the net result is the same. These seniors are being taken care of by involved Chadults who do not perceive their work as a burden or a chore.

While many good relationships between parents and Chadults exist, it is also important to remember that sometimes things look rosier from the outside than they do to those who actually live them. The grass, indeed, often looks greener on the other side.

Terry came from a very dysfunctional home. Her mother was mentally ill and her father was too scatterbrained to pay much attention. She had very little in the way of parenting and the establishment of boundaries so necessary to a youngster in the formative years.

In her teen years Terry met a friend who seemed to come from a home invented in Hollywood.

Eleanor the mother, was beautiful. Winston, the father, was handsome and worldly. Her friend was so pretty. How Terry clung to these three perfect people! She would go home and her mother's ravaged face would sicken her. She could not help but compare it with her friend's mother's beautifully made-up face, perfect figure, and glamorous clothing.

As the years went on, Terry spent more and more time at her friend's. They were inseparable. They shared every thought and secret. Her friend would tell her, "I love you best," despite being surrounded by boyfriends.

Eventually the two young women got married, and then there was a foursome. During all those years Terry never gave an inch to her parents. Everything good and beautiful was at her friend's home. She even called her friend's parents Mom and Dad.

But, just as if this were a fable rather than a true story, Terry was given a shattering blow. Her "best friend" had been having a long-standing affair with Terry's husband. Her friend's mother, a kind and loving woman as well as the epitome of perfect womanhood, had developed a prescription-drug addiction.

Her friend's father had turned mean and unkind in his later years.

It was then, finally, that Terry took a good long look at her own people. Certainly her mother was still mentally ill and her father was still scatterbrained. But now, after all her illusions had been so dreadfully shattered, Terry could begin to understand that her mother needed compassion, not contempt. Her father needed to be understood because he lived with a woman with whom there could be no relationship. Terry began to look deeper and in their final years gave her parents filial duty and care.

"I learned that old saying that all that glitters is not gold," she says. "I learned it about my friend and her family. They were not living a lie. They were just who they were. I was living the lie. I had the illusions and the fantasy pictures in my mind. Once I got past all of that I was able to be a reasonably caring daughter. I had stopped comparing that family to mine. At least I was now dealing with reality—even though that reality was painful."

But most of all Terry expresses gratitude for her ability to demonstrate caring during her parents' final years.

Terry's experience was different from that of most Chadults, because she had felt the loss of a parent when she was much younger. At an early age she watched mental deterioration in her mother. Her mother had long been unable to interact with her.

This is much like the loss that Chadults experience—only they experience it at an age when they do not need their mother for sustenance and maturation.

Once they see how the aging process brings about loss of

physical and mental abilities, Chadults are prone to going back into their own childhood experiences to try to learn how to deal with their parents.

The difficulty with this is that many Chadults cannot draw on personal experience as Terry could. They are walking on unfamiliar ground, and each step can feel as if it might land them in quicksand. They have never seen their parents child-like and vulnerable. They have not seen Mom or Dad needing rescue before.

It is possible they felt the need to rescue when Mom or Dad became widowed. They saw how vulnerable their surviving parent had become. But, if the parent was healthy, they worked together and the Chadult helped to restructure the surviving parent's life.

Even that is a role reversal. Helping Dad restructure his life is probably difficult and unsettling for most Chadults. After all, Dad was the provider. In older generations he was the prime decision-maker. He was the head of the house.

Children may even have been taught by their mothers to "sit straight at the table when your father is here." Or "speak when you are spoken to when your father is home." Or "make certain your father has enough chicken before you start taking for yourself."

Now that Mom is dead, the Chadult is thrust in the role of helping his once-powerful Dad.

Surprisingly, this is accomplished effectively in most cir-cumstances when a parent is widowed. Helping Dad does not work quite as smoothly when he begins to deteriorate, even though the Chadult must similarly take control in this unfamil-iar position.

Chadults often feel a lack of certainty about their decision-making and need reassurance that they are "doing the right thing."

Many gerontologists, social workers, and support groups are available to help people who need positive reinforcement about what they are doing. It is wise to avail yourself of such help.

If the Chadult and the parent were not close in the past, there are many people who perhaps will think, "too little, too late." And in some instances this could well be true, especially if the Chadult allows himself to be flogged for not being attentive over the years or allows himself to feel guilty for each argument, even the ones started by his parent.

One thing is certain: only the person who lived the experience can excuse himself from the guilt he feels. He alone understands the underlying reasons for his lack of attentiveness. He alone can make the choice to change his behavior or decide he can live with things as they are.

Therapy can be useful. It can help us to learn things about our behavior that might give us the option to alter how we act. When we know and understand our own backgrounds and the things that formed us and our thinking, we are better equipped to make decisions about how to treat our parents. Being a Chadult gives us the right of choice. But it is always wise to remember that long after our parents are dead, those choices will remain with us, as will guilt about our actions or freedom from such painful feelings.

The poet John Greenleaf Whittier wrote, "Of all sad things of tongue or pen, / The saddest are these: 'It might have been!' "

Ricky felt a lurching in her stomach every time she was about to visit her elderly father, Howard. He had always been a distant person, who never showed warmth toward his only daughter. Did he even feel any? Ricky had no way of knowing. While her mother was alive Ricky would discuss this question with her but she never received an answer that satisfied her. She always felt there was evasion. If truth were to be told she never even knew how her mother felt about her.

Now Howard had suffered a stroke and was going through rehabilitation at the nursing home where he lived. There had never been any question of his moving in with Ricky and her family. The rejection had gone too far and too deep for her even to consider it.

But out of some strong sense of duty, Ricky visited Howard several times a week. The visits were never pleasant. Even before his stroke, her father would sit there with downcast eyes, saying little and forcing Ricky to initiate whatever conversation they exchanged.

After each visit she would shake her head and once again consider the puzzle of her father. Here she was, a Chadult with a loving husband and grown children. She had a rewarding career as an accountant. Everything was in place, yet sadness always overtook her when she came to see her father.

She knew there would be people who would say it was the setting, the nursing home. But she knew better. It was nothing like that at all. The sadness went deeper. It went all the way back to her youth.

Ricky understood that no amount of therapy to help her father regain his physical being after the stroke would make him a man she could turn to and ask a question of with the certainty that she would receive a considered, loving answer.

Ricky would think of her friends, both those whose parents were still alert and on the go and those whose parents had died and were mourned by their adult children.

She would shake her head and think, "What a thing to envy. Someone who mourns their dead mother or father!"

Ricky's depression is typical of a Chadult who has long had a difficult or distant relationship with a parent. It is hard to forget all that waste, all that might have been, all that we wish we could have shaken out of our mothers or fathers, all the spontaneous hugs that never happened, the indifference to our successes, the sense of feeling unloved . . . being unloved without understanding why, the hurt of seeing a more favored child, the memories of being ignored when we ran forward to hug a father or mother, the sense of living our lives on shifting sands because there was no solid floor beneath us to hold us steady. These are the roots of depression in many people.

Often our troubles are compounded when we marry. Frequently we do not choose mates who will help us build strong positive relationships during our adult years. Rather, many mental health experts believe we select partners who resemble the parent with whom we have unresolved issues. Thus we give ourselves another opportunity to work through those issues and have them come out correctly. We want a happy ending.

But many people, like Ricky, are able to understand the realities about their background and come to at least a partial resolution.

It took Ricky years of therapy to understand that no amount of effort on her part could alter her father or their relationship. Howard would always be aloof and apparently indifferent to any overture she might make. He had grown up in an unhappy home where there was no nurturing and had never learned the art of giving of himself. Therapy enabled Ricky to find a loving mate and build a loving relationship with her children.

Despite these positive parts of her life, when she visited her father out of duty, she always left with a sense of sadness and the knowledge that the next visit would be no different.

Todd, her husband, finally made her realize that her visits to her father were carrying over into their home life and making the entire family unhappy because she was so depressed. She discovered then that, although therapy had helped her in many ways, not everything has a solution.

She learned also that not everything has a happy ending. This was the time when Ricky needed her family to understand her feelings and needs. She took the time to explain to them that there would never be a time when her father would care overly that she was there. She visited him for her own needs and hoped it helped him along the way. Once her family understood this they were kinder when she returned from the nursing home.

On the other hand there are parents and children who have extraordinarily close relationships.

Robert and his father, Michael, were fishing buddies, partners in business, and traveling companions. They were more than father and son. The two men liked each other. They were friends.

One snowy December evening the father was returning home from a party when an oncoming car skidded across the road and slammed into him. Michael was near death for more than a week and his recovery was minimal. He stayed on life-support systems for a month before he died.

During that month Robert visited his father daily. As often as possible he would stand by the bedside and talk to his father as if he could understand and hear. Occasionally he would read the newspaper to him, but more often he would remind the older man of trips they had taken together and tell him the news of their business. But it was all to no avail.

Robert would leave the intensive care unit with tears streaming down his cheeks. At first he would try to cover them because "Grown men don't cry." But then a nurse stopped him and they spoke for a while.

"Why are you crying?" she asked.

"My dad and I are very close. We always did everything together. Now I'm running the business alone. I'm hurting inside. My guts feel as if they're burning. And even worse, I'm depressed. I realize I'll never be able to ask him about anything again. This is the end of the line. It hurts."

The nurse heard him out and nodded. "But just don't be ashamed of how you feel. You have a right to be depressed. You need not hide those tears. They are honest and they are for a person you love. How lucky he is that someone cares so deeply. We don't always see that here."

Diane is another devoted Chadult. Her primary interest in life is her family: her husband, her children, and her mother.

Despite being a grandmother herself and a charming and gracious woman who is much sought after socially, she spends many hours visiting with her mother, whom she calls her closest girlfriend. The two shop together, lunch together, visit infant grandchildren together. When the northern winter gets harsh Diane and as many of her family members as are able head south for warmer weather. Her mother is always part of that group.

Now her mother, Sylvia, is getting on in years and walks a little less steadily, but she is treated just as she always was. Frequently she accompanies her daughter and son-in-law to dinner on Saturday night. She insists on maintaining her own apartment but knows she is welcome in her daughter's home at any time, or for that matter, in her grandchildren's homes.

Diane knows she is seeing the beginnings of loss in her mother: "There are some days when she is not as quick mentally as she used to be. I see it and recognize it. But when she has a good day I try to use that time wisely by discussing with her what it is she would like should she become incapacitated. She is very willing to share her thoughts with me. I understand that this sort of discussion is rare. But I would never want to do anything she would be unhappy with, and the only way I can be certain of her wishes is if she tells me. As close as we are, I would never presume to second-guess her on an issue as big as how she wants to live out her final years. I love her very much, but I can't read her mind."

Because many Chadults have very full, rich lives, and because they are busy making decisions and functioning with a certain amount of power, they may spend little time thinking about the fact that their parents are aging. The idea that something vital like illness or age will not be in their control can be painful and depressing. Aging makes them acknowledge that there are times when all of us are powerless.

The aphorist Charles C. Colton spoke of power with a sense of warning. He said, "Power will intoxicate the best hearts, as wine the strongest heads. No man is wise enough nor good enough to be trusted with unlimited power."

All too often Chadults forget this. None of us should have unlimited power. We can hope and plan and pray, but we are only able to do so much, and some things are just not in our control.

Unfortunately, many in the geriatric helping field say that powerlessness creates a sense of separation between parent and Chadult. When a Chadult sees there is nothing that can be done to jog the memory of someone suffering from Alzheimer's, or help a paralyzed stroke victim, or ease the pain of a parent dying of cancer who wishes to remain alert, he will sometimes withdraw rather than face the slow deterioration of the vital person he once knew.

Adele owns a large travel agency with fifty or more employees, including two personal secretaries. She runs a tight organization, allowing little room for error. She does not tolerate mistakes easily or kindly. Some former employees see her organization as a solid training ground from which to move on to happier work environments.

Adele has never married. Her agency has been her life. Her father died when she was in high school, but he left both Adele and Greta, her mother, amply provided for, so her mother never worked outside the home, and Adele was able to complete her college education as the family had always planned.

Greta took great pride in Adele's scholastic and business achievements. She loved telling people how kind her daughter was to her, how she sent her on trips. It did not matter that many of these excursions cost Adele nothing; it was the idea that Adele thought of sending her mother that mattered.

Indeed, Adele did care for her mother. She admired the way her mother conducted herself, the way she looked when she came to the office to visit. She liked the friends her mother chose. At the back of her mind Adele always thought that if the day came when she retired she would like to emulate her mother.

Despite her toughness as a boss, Adele was an involved and caring daughter.

Then, inevitably, Greta began to show her age. Her step was not as steady, she began having fender-benders, she occasionally forgot luncheon dates with her daughter or other friends, she did not always get the punch line of a joke as quickly as she had done in earlier days.

She was getting older.

Adele saw what was happening and began looking for resources to slow the aging process. She had her secretaries call around the country looking for the best clinics, the most knowledgeable geriatric specialists, seeking the advice of the finest medical and mental health professionals that money could buy.

She was determined that her mother should feel and be better. But, sadly, it was all to no avail. The deterioration continued. Greta fell and needed a walker. She was no longer able to drive, so Adele hired a driver for her. She no longer showed any interest in lunching with friends, and more and more quickly she began to forget the names of objects and people. Adele was told her mother had Alzheimer's disease, so the deterioration was irreversible.

Adele hired staff for around-the-clock care in her mother's luxurious apartment. This worked for a while. And Adele made it a point to visit three to four times a week, even if only briefly.

But Greta reached a point where she needed the more specialized care that can best be given in the Alzheimer's disease unit of a nursing home. Adele was appalled. All the resources in the world had not stopped the progression of the illness or kept her mother from a nursing home.

It had been many years since Adele had cried, but she now found herself crying frequently, filled as she was with sadness and facing the evidence of her own powerlessness.

"I wanted to do so much for her," she says. "I am a powerful woman and have the money and clout to make things happen. But I couldn't do anything for her. It hurt me and surprised me. I hadn't realized I was so vulnerable. This was beyond anything I could change or make better."

Adele joined a support group and shared her experience. She had never dreamed that *she* would attend such a gathering. But the nursing home had organized the group and the social worker had called to invite her after noticing that her visits had dropped off.

Adele admits, "I had stopped going as often because I felt it was useless. She didn't know me half the time and talked gibberish part of the time. I just couldn't bear to see her like that, so I came to see her less and less."

What Adele learned at the meeting was how important it was to continue the visits. Even if her mother could not always appreciate them, there *were* moments when her mind was clear.

There was another reason to keep visiting. That reason had to do with Adele herself. There would come a day in the future when her mother would die and Adele, who had no siblings, would be left with no immediate family. The visits were for Adele's future peace of mind, for those days when she would need to comfort herself with the knowledge that she had indeed done all she could for her mother.

The urge to pull away, to withdraw, is something that seems to be particularly strong in highly successful people. People who are used to being in control know how to act when they can exert that control. Powerlessness is at best uncomfortable and at worst something from which many people run.

Chadults need to understand they run at their own risk. At risk is how they will perceive themselves for the rest of their lives!

There is a saying that adversity introduces man to himself.

Most Chadults who have to face changes and difficulties and distress over their parents come to know themselves quite well.

They go through all the painful stages of their parents' deterioration. The stages can vary in length, intensity, and sequence. They go through denial, unwilling to accept what is happening. They deal with anger, and if they are wise they conquer it and use it as an incentive to go forward with their lives. They are generally faced with guilt in one form or another. While often guilt does not go away, it does ease with time. They handle depression and the painful sadness it can bring. They meet powerlessness and do not like it. Some, indeed, meet if for the first time. But when there is no alternative they have to accept it.

Many mental health experts claim that it takes several years before a Chadult feels back in control after the death of a parent when powerlessness is a major factor.

The issue of powerlessness is of great moment when a loved one dies. There is the sense that somehow, somewhere, one should have been able to save the special person. However, there is the reality of knowing there will come a day, in the *normal* sequence of events, when our parents will precede us in death. If, during their lifetime, we have helped them to the best of our ability and done what the Chadult and parent mutually feel is the right thing, there can be a gentle letting go, an acceptance that precludes being trapped in the issue of powerlessness.

Since powerlessness equates with loss of control, it can be of comfort to know that a time will come when the Chadult *will* be back in control.

For those people still experiencing great difficulty in coming to terms with a parent's death, support groups in hospitals, nursing homes, and senior centers can be invaluable. Do not overlook this resource.

Above all, as our parents age and we see the future, we must try to do what will not only make them feel better but also help us to heal ourselves afterward.

There is nothing in these stages of loss that is beyond our ability to cope. This does not mean there will be no pain, because very often there is great pain.

When we see our parents deteriorating, we feel great sadness, not only because we see them going downward but also because they are once again showing us a path that most of us will follow. They are doing what they did all our lives: showing us and teaching us and letting us learn from them what was appropriate and what was folly.

If we are willing to view this with a clear eye and open mind, we can offer our own children a legacy. We are free to determine what that legacy will be: the way we treat our parents shows them how we wish to be treated.

It is not realistic to offer more than we can deliver. But by being realistic and knowing that most people go through most of the stages of denial and anger and guilt and depression and powerlessness and weakness, we can serve as teachers.

Diane, who is so devoted to her mother, finds that her daughters treat her in the same manner. She is loved and respected and valued.

When the time comes that Diane's mother is incapacitated or dies, there will certainly be great sorrow. But an entire family will be able to derive comfort from knowing how their mother and grandmother and mother-in-law was treated.

In their very busy lives they always made time for her.

When we determine how we will treat aging parents, it is important to know that *we* are doing the determining. We are not sliding into a role.

Certainly, Mom or Dad can suddenly become ill and lose faculties, but Chadults must always remember that the decision about how to handle the change is a choice. It is the choice of the Chadult.

Understanding some of the dynamics of loss may enable Chadults to make better choices and thus feel more comfortable about how they dealt with the situation.

Chapter 6

FAMILY

———◇———

It is characteristic of man that he
alone has any sense of good and evil,
or just and unjust, and the like, and the
association of living things who have
this sense makes a family and a state.

—Aristotle, *Politics,* 1

S ince so much of society has changed during the past half
century, our definition of what constitutes a family may
well need updating.

Sometimes that family can reflect the traditional: birth
mother and father, and children, who are now Chadults.

A family may also include stepparents and stepsiblings,
who are either of long standing or new to the unit.

Since transiency is such a major factor in our ever changing world, a neighbor or friend may be as loving as any family member.

Some foster parents who raised children for years maintain a close and loving relationship with them.

Sometimes mothers and fathers have felt unable to raise a newborn infant and have opted for adoption. Frequently, in later years, their longing to know the child is overwhelming and they seek and find the son or daughter. Sometimes the son or daughter feels this same intensity. In either event, if the biological parent is aged and needy, what does the Chadult who was given up for adoption feel? Is there any sense of wishing to care for the parent?

While in many families, the mother-in-law–daughter-in-law discord is a myth, there are times when the conflict is very real. In such instances, how can Chadults better interact when their parents are in need?

Since many gay and lesbian couples are becoming more public about their relationship, are other family members supportive? Can long-standing angers be set aside when one of the partners is aging and needs help?

Should a stepparent become ill, will the Chadult be able to set aside feelings of resentment and treat a parent's spouse kindly?

The stepparent is another example of how the family unit has changed. As we can see, there are many different components that can make up the relationship that was once the exclusive realm of the "traditional" family.

In each of these circumstances there may be Chadults who are trying to find their way.

Family structures today are increasingly complex. They are complex when a parent remarries during a youngster's childhood. They are equally complex when the parent of a Chadult remarries.

Estelle, who was in her mid-sixties, had been a widow for a dozen years. She had been collecting Social Security and living on a savings plan she and her husband had established many years earlier.

Jerome had been a widower for just over a year when he and Estelle met at a senior singles event. They liked each other. He appreciated her sense of humor and how well she had maintained herself physically. She appreciated his warmth and his willingness to try new things.

To her children, their courtship seemed very quick.

"Why don't you take your time and go slower? Really get to know the man," her daughter, Lisa, would say again and again.

Estelle would always answer that her daughter could not comprehend that when you are sixty-five taking your time is not a priority.

"I don't have endless years ahead of me," she would say.

After six months Estelle and Jerome invited her two children and his son out to dinner and announced they were getting married in two weeks.

The Chadults and their spouses looked at one another openmouthed. The six of them were meeting for the first time and suddenly they were going to be family!

"What in the world are these two old people doing?" was the thought that ran through all the Chadults' minds. "How can they know they are doing the right thing after only six months?"

Estelle's daughter finally voiced what they were all feeling: "Look, I think you seem like a nice man, Jerome, but do you really know my mother well enough to want to marry her? Do you know Jerome well enough to want to marry him, Mom?"

Estelle, who had been nervous about this first meeting and their announcement, became angry:

"You are not my mother. I am your mother! I still have my mind and I know what I am doing. We are going to get married. If you want to come to our wedding, you can. If you don't . . . well, you won't!"

Lisa was taken aback by this forcefulness. This was not the meek, submissive woman she had gotten comfortable with since her mother became a widow. She began to remember how forthright her mother had always been during her growing-up years. It was only since her father died that this meekness had taken over.

When she recalled the differences in her mother's behavior before her widowhood and after, she grudgingly had to admit that this forceful woman was far more attractive. She had more character and more carriage. In truth, this was the mother who raised her.

She saw that her brother, Scott, was about to object and she shook her head quickly.

"Look, Mom, you raised us and you did it with a pretty level head. I've got to think you still have that head, and if this is what you want I'll certainly be at your wedding."

Her mother smiled a look of appreciation at her daughter. Her son looked a bit surprised, but then he reached his hand out to Jerome and congratulated him.

Jerome's son, Dale, seeing this, was not to be outdone. He, too, shook hands with his father and reached for Estelle's hand and held it warmly.

Certainly, there would be many questions about practical issues, but the first hurdle had been overcome because Estelle demonstrated her strength and her certainty that she was doing the right thing.

Fortunately for her, her daughter remembered that strength, and its familiarity made her comfortable.

While many newly connected families do not work as smoothly, Estelle and Jerome's Chadults saw a fait accompli and were wise enough to fall in line. They even got together to plan the small reception following the wedding.

After the honeymoon the new couple came back to a new apartment they had rented because both agreed they wanted a fresh start.

When they invited their families over for the first time, Jerome stood up and proposed a toast to his bride and all of their children. "You will never know the depths of my loneliness after your mother died," he said to Dale. "Nearly fifty years of my life and then an empty house. Thank you all for making this new chapter a happy one. I'll always remember and honor your mother just as Estelle has honored her husband. You can be certain of that."

Then he stopped for a moment, looked at everyone assembled, and smiled. "We are not dummies. If we didn't know how good our lives had been we wouldn't be going to try for a second marriage!"

His son laughed, although he had felt as if his mother was being betrayed. "I guess you're right. Your getting married again is sort of a compliment to Mother . . . in a strange way, that is."

Some Chadults believe they were told of parents' marriage plans completely inappropriately.

Ann says she and her brothers were not treated sympathetically when their father decided to remarry. "He waited until we had all come back to our hometown for the unveiling of Mother's tombstone. After the ceremony was over we all went to a restaurant feeling pretty somber. My dad stood up and took a woman's hand in his. None of us had ever met her. He told us she was going to be his new wife. They were getting married within the month!"

She still speaks with fury at the memory. "Here we had just placed a marker over our mother's grave and he was announcing his remarriage. He could have waited until another time to tell us! Certainly the unveiling was the wrong time."

Ann says that though it was completely unfair to do so, all the siblings took an immediate dislike to the woman. "We were angry at Dad, but it was easier to vent our fury on her."

Chadults are frequently fairly resilient. But they need courtesy from their parents. Ann's story is not unique. Many mothers and fathers have displayed equal insensitivity in their eagerness to remarry.

However, adult children need to understand the urgency their parents may be feeling about being alone. Balance is always necessary in such situations.

The old person's need to move quickly has other far-reaching implications. It can lead to bad judgment in choosing a mate, but as long as Mom or Dad is mentally alert and able to decide things they have the right to do so.

Sometimes the best we as Chadults can do is to be loving and supportive. If things fall apart, do not say, "I told you so." Without question some of these marriages will fall apart, and the added hurt can be devastating.

On the other hand, when a Chadult has an open mind it is possible to see beauty emerge from chaos.

Stan remembers all too well the stormy house in which he was raised. His mother, Audrey, constantly berated his father, Nathan. He did not earn enough money. He did not act friendly enough socially. He dressed badly. Nothing he did was quite good enough.

When Nathan died Stan stood at the graveside and shook his head. Well, at least the nagging was over for Dad now, he thought.

Within months Audrey announced she was remarrying. Stan, a passive man in his early fifties, simply shrugged. He asked his mother only once if she wasn't rushing things a bit, and she told him to mind his own business.

Ironically, the man his mother was marrying seemed to resemble his father. But as the months went by Stan began to notice a change in his mother. She had somehow blossomed. She spoke to her new husband lovingly. The two held hands continually. They always sat side by side and even whispered to one another, sharing private things.

Stan could not remember his mother ever kissing his father, yet here she was kissing and holding hands and showing great love and affection.

The effect on Stan was unusual. Rather than resent this change in his mother, he grew to enjoy her more than he had in all his years. She was open and affectionate and obviously happy. The change brought out a feeling of love in him for her that he had not previously experienced.

Sometimes love can have such power.

Chadults sometimes have to come to terms with the idea that the person their parent chooses to marry is from a different faith or a different background or economic group.

One widow, Bethany, who is part of the country-club set, has wanted to remarry for the past five years but, despite her wealth, has dated only occasionally. Henry was one man she went out with five or six times before introducing him to her daughters. Their response was not positive.

"But, Mom, look at his car. It's small and it isn't even new," one daughter, DeeDee, said.

"His clothes are no better," said Lindsay, the other. "He looks disheveled. How can you take him to the club like that?"

Her children were coming from the secure position of having their spouses and children and home lives intact. They could not begin to know the depths of her aloneness.

But she heard them. She looked at Henry and assessed his car and his clothing and, yes, even his table manners and decided her daughters were right. This, despite how she enjoyed his quick wit and dancing with him.

She is still alone.

In such situations, Chadults would do well to think twice before casting judgments on their parent's choices. They are not walking in Mom or Dad's moccasins, and they should remember that this person raised them. This person is older and may be wiser than they. It's Mom or Dad's life and a Chadult doesn't have the right to parent when he or she is the child.

Pat, a social worker, was very unhappy with her mother, Corinne's, remarriage. "She couldn't have used any thought. He just doesn't fit in with our family or her friends. He's from a different background."

Right before the wedding, the Chadult took her mother out to lunch. Corinne knew something big was coming because of the emphasis on this lunch for just the two of them.

When Pat spoke her piece about her future stepfather not fitting in, her mother took her hand and smiled at her with a look of love. "Don't you think I haven't noticed? I'm not that blind. But I've weighed how empty my life is without my own person and I decided the trade-off was worth it. I think I'm going to be very happy."

She thanked her daughter for her concern, thereby wisely averting a confrontation.

As time went by, Gordon, the new mate, although never quite fitting hand-in-glove, became a fun grandfather to the children and a nice person to invite to dinner along with Corinne.

By averting a confrontation, the mother did not allow passions to grow strong. She was loving but firm with her daughter—and, most important, she retained her role as mother.

Of course, there are people at the opposite end of the financial scale from the woman who was of the country-club set. These are the people like June, a woman whose husband, Roger, died when she was fifty-seven. He left no money, their home was a rented apartment, and she would not be eligible for Social Security for some years.

June had been a homemaker all her life and was not trained for the business world. She could not ask her children for money they did not have.

She married Timothy, the first man who asked her.

Bruce, her Chadult son, did not like him. When he asked June why she had chosen that particular man, his mother laughed.

"You say 'chosen' as if there were a long line of men waiting to marry me," she said. "It just doesn't work that way, son. There are so many single women out there, and so few decent men who don't drink or gamble away their paychecks. I did the best I could."

Bruce went no further. He knew he could offer his mother nothing financially; if she felt taken care of by Timothy, then he had no right to interfere.

He understood that he was not walking in her moccasins. But he would never know that she felt her very survival depended upon marrying this man who had a steady income and could keep a roof over her head.

Sometimes Chadults are not clear in their own minds about why they object to a remarriage of a parent. The objection is not always as clear-cut as "It's too soon," "So-and-So doesn't fit in." Sometimes Chadults worry about Mother's annuity ending upon her remarriage.

And, yes, sometimes Chadults even feel their inheritance is being threatened.

There is yet another area Chadults consider. They frequently are worried about who will be responsible if their parent or the new mate becomes ill.

One couple who married late in life found themselves in a great deal of difficulty over this issue.

Lorraine and Peter enjoyed eight wonderful years together before the aging process took hold. Lorraine broke a hip, and shortly thereafter she began to lose much of her alertness. Peter was devastated. He had come to love this woman of his later years with all his heart and he saw that he was losing her.

Lorraine had one daughter, Amy, who had not been delighted about the marriage. She came to their home and began issuing orders about how her mother should be handled.

Peter, a man in his late seventies, knew he would need help to care for his wife, but Amy, made him very angry. "You are bossing me around as if I were a child!" he said after one of her onslaughts in his home.

"She is my mother and I want to take care of her," the daughter retorted angrily.

Both Peter and the daughter were fortunate that his son, Kevin, came in just at this point.

Kevin had grown quite fond of Lorraine, and Amy knew

this. He offered to sit down with both of them and help organize a care plan so that both would feel part of a team. He also suggested calling in a professional social worker who could help them work out the plan.

When Amy and Peter realized that they both wanted the same results they allowed reason to prevail. They called the hospital where Lorraine was a patient and made an appointment with the social worker, who was very helpful.

Her suggestions were well received. And during the remainder of the year Lorraine lived, Amy and Peter developed a friendship that lasted until he died several years later.

Of course, there are many circumstances in which things do not run as smoothly. Sometimes Chadults from one side of the marriage feel they are being taken advantage of by the children of the other side. Sometimes Chadults are unhappy when the new spouse becomes ill and requires a great deal of their own parent's energy.

But if two people can find some years to enjoy together late in life, perhaps Chadults can look at this with a kind eye and the understanding that despite the changes we've seen in society's structures, people who are older still generally think of life as going two by two just as it was on Noah's Ark.

Sometimes non–family members can be extraordinarily caring. There is an old legend about one such neighbor.

In the year 1306 King Philip IV of France expelled all Jews from his kingdom. He gave them two days to leave. Any Jew found in the kingdom after that would be put to death.

Because the time was so limited most people were forced to leave without selling their belongings. They had to depart with nothing but what they could carry.

One of the Jews was a jeweler whose stock included many precious stones. He was afraid to take them with him because he feared they would be confiscated.

He went to his neighbor, who was not Jewish, and asked him to guard the treasure. "Someday the king will change his mind. When that happens I will return and claim my jewels."

The neighbor promised to guard them well. The Jew left France and wandered with all the others to find a new refuge.

Many years later the king died and a successor altered the policy toward the exiled Jews. Upon hearing word of this many of them returned to their native land.

The first thing the jeweler did, of course, was to go to his neighbor's home to greet him and regain his property, but the neighbor did not live there any longer.

When he went to other people in the area they told him the neighbor had lost all his money and had been forced to move to a desolate area outside the city.

When the wanderer heard this he felt certain his fortune was gone. After all, if the neighbor was destitute it was only to be expected that he would use the jewels for his own survival. Although he was saddened he set out on foot to find his neighbor.

He reached a place where poverty was rampant. When he found the man he was shocked. The once-proud gentleman was thin and in rags, sitting on a crate in a room that did not even hold a bed.

The tattered man recognized his friend and uttered a shout of delight. He then jumped up, reached into the crate, and handed the wanderer the jewels.

"I have guarded your treasure carefully. I knew you would return someday," he said.

"How could you have done such a thing? You are destitute. Why didn't you use the jewels to buy food or shelter?"

"I couldn't have taken something that belonged to you. There were many times I even thought of killing myself but could not because I needed to take care of your treasure."

The wanderer was moved to tears. "I am grateful that you did not take your life and that you waited for me to return. You are better than a brother to me, and half of what is in that bag is yours."

The two men once again bought homes side by side and lived out their lives with great caring for one another.

Indeed, a friend or a neighbor can be that close.

One Chadult, Keith, was greatly chagrined by this sort of relationship. His mother, Lenore, and her friend Judy had been inseparable for over half a century, since they were children. Both women were now widows.

One day Lenore suffered a stroke and after her hospital stay was brought home to recuperate. Whether in the hospital or at home, Keith was never able to see his mother alone. Judy was always there. She would hover over his mother, feed her, massage her hands and feet, and comb her hair. In fact, there was nothing she left undone.

Every time Keith arrived for a visit, everything was in place; the woman was completely cared for—and he was angered over his inability to have any privacy with his own mother.

He would go home after these visits and tell his wife, Idie, of his frustration. She would remind him that they would have had to hire nurses or spend all that time with his mother themselves. Since both had busy careers it was not possible for them to give her that amount of time.

Eventually Idie told him he needed to talk with Judy. He needed to be gentlemanly but he certainly needed to share what he was feeling.

Privately, she felt that if her mother-in-law died it would be very sad for her husband to feel so pushed aside.

When he visited Lenore the following evening, Judy was sitting there brushing his mother's hair and crying. When he saw this he walked over to her and put an arm around her shoulder and nudged her toward the kitchen where they could talk privately.

"Has anything happened?" Keith asked.

"No," Judy replied. "But I can see she is getting weaker. I'm afraid I'm going to lose her."

"So am I," said Keith. "That's why I need you to help me. You see her all day long, and you're alone with her most of that time. I only have a few hours in the evening, and I'd like to spend that time just with her."

He gave her a hug and again told her he needed her help and hoped she understood.

Judy was startled. It had never occurred to her that she allowed him no time alone.

"But why have you waited so long?" she asked. "You should have told me earlier. I would never do anything to hurt you. I've known you all your life."

He hugged her again and thanked her. He learned then that as his mother further deteriorated he had a special ally. Equally important, he discovered the value of speaking up about an issue in an appropriate manner.

Through the years we have seen splendid television programs about foster parents who offer loving intervention and safety for a young person who is frightened and feels alone at a time of great crisis.

Rose was proud of the fact that she had "fostered" more than 120 children over some thirty years. Some of the children came to her because a parent had died suddenly. Others came to her because courts ordered them removed from unsafe homes. Still others came because parents were divorcing and neither wanted the burden of raising the children.

In any event these children all were in great need. Rose was an extraordinary woman, who was able to offer wisdom and love and a warm place for "the kids."

She would bathe them and feed them and make certain her own children were part of the process of caring. There were even times she battled with social workers because she felt one of "the kids" was being removed from her care too soon. She generally lost those battles, so she thought poorly of social service agencies.

What she did do when she believed youngsters were being prematurely removed was give them her telephone number and ask them to call and stay in touch. Quite a few of them did.

Many of the agency workers would have been surprised to know that the foster children remained in regular contact with Rose. As young adults with more freedom, "the kids" frequently visited and spent hours talking over problems and recalling events from their earlier youth.

Rose enjoyed these visits greatly because they also made it a point to talk with the new "kids."

"They were the greatest help because they knew how it felt," she said. "They told the 'kids' they could trust me and gave them examples from their own experience that reinforced this."

Because her natural children all lived out of town, when Rose became ill the "kids" argued over whose home would be best for her to live in.

Some had gone on to achieve financial success despite their uncertain beginnings. Others had limited funds but could care for her because they worked at home.

When her daughter, Toby, came to town and offered to take her home with her Rose started to laugh.

"Everyone wants me. Everyone wants to take care of me. But no one asked me what I wanted. Well, I'll tell you anyhow. I want to go to a nursing home. They'll take good care of me there and everyone can come and visit and when they are tired of me they can go home. That's what *I* want."

Toby tried arguing with her, but Rose was adamant. She knew her own mind. "I've raised a hundred and twenty children and by this time I think I know what is best for me. I am the parent and this is my decision."

Toby reluctantly let all the "kids" know her mother's decision. Each felt some discomfort. She had done so much for them. Now they were Chadults. They wanted to repay her and now they had a chance. Didn't Rose understand?

Toby said she completely understood. But she would not go against her mother's wishes.

"Let's all figure out a visiting schedule and make sure we stick to it," she suggested. "That way we're doing what she wants but still staying involved in her care."

Although unhappy, they finally agreed.

These people kept their agreement. Rose never had a time where she wished someone, anyone, would come to visit. The Chadults had a schedule and regardless of how busy their lives became, there was always time to visit Auntie Rose. They came with their own children and their spouses to visit the woman they believed had saved them at the time of their greatest fear and peril.

When she died several years after entering the nursing home, the number of mourners who called themselves her "kids" startled the funeral director!

Toby watched the look of bewilderment on his face for a few moments, and then she took pity on him and explained the situation.

Pews across the entire front of the chapel were cordoned off to allow the "kids" to sit together as mourners.

During Rose's time in the nursing home many of the Chadults felt they simply were not doing enough, but other residents of the home would marvel at the number of visitors Rose received and at the love they all showed her.

There are varying reasons parents give up their children for adoption. Sometimes they are too young to raise them in a responsible manner. Sometimes they simply are not interested in having the youngster impinge on their lives. Sometimes the birth parents or mother lives in dreadful grinding poverty.

In many cases the child given up for adoption is then raised by two parents, possibly with other siblings and generally in a financially secure home. Often the child has the opportunity to go to good schools and become a contributing member of the community.

For many adopted children this is enough. The people who raised them and took care of them through chicken pox and measles are their real parents. But there are other adoptees who, as adults, feel a restless inner craving to know the man and woman who gave them life.

Sometimes the search can take years.

Shelby, who was a college student, wanted desperately to find his birth mother. Elizabeth, his adoptive mother, knew and honored his need. She gave him all the information she had, which was scanty, but she also told him about a person she had seen on television whose whole career was to seek out missing parents and children.

Since Shelby went on his quest with his parents' blessing,

he did not feel he was betraying them; they were secure in his love and he in theirs.

He ultimately found his birth mother, Wanda, who was dying of cancer. She cried endlessly when she saw him. She repeatedly told him how guilty she felt for having given him up.

He had been prepared for this response, but not for her illness. He called Elizabeth, his adoptive mother, and told her the circumstances. He explained that his biological mother had no one in the world who cared about her. He wanted to stay in the vicinity for the short time she had left. He asked his adoptive mother how she would feel if he switched colleges for a year or so in order to complete the task of helping his birth mother. She said she would have to talk to his father to discuss his feelings about the intense involvement and also his changing schools.

Meanwhile the young Chadult spent hours that first day asking Wanda about her background. He discovered there was much cancer in her family, which disquieted him greatly. His birth father was dead; he had gotten drunk the night Shelby was born and had been hit by a car as he staggered across a busy street.

Wanda shared openly what she knew about the man and his family history. All the while the Chadult was writing down information that could at some later date save his life.

When he saw how ill this woman was, he decided not to let matters rest with his father. He called his mother back and told her *he* had made the decision. This was something he had to do. If she wanted to, she was welcome to come and visit him and even meet his birth mother. But he needed to stay there because she was so ill.

"The problem is, you raised me with a sense of responsibility and now it's popping up all over the place, Mom," he told her. "I just can't walk away."

Elizabeth, his adoptive mother, felt tears stinging her eyes when he said this. She nodded, although he could not see her.

"Of course," she said. "You have no choice. Daddy and I *will* come see you, and maybe even meet the woman who gave us our greatest treasure."

Surprisingly, she was as good as her word and both she and her husband did come to visit. They met the dying woman and saw how empty and pitiful her life was. When they looked at their handsome son they could only feel gratitude that this woman had given them such a gift.

Elizabeth sent clothing and food and stayed in close telephone contact with her son once she returned home.

When Wanda died the Chadult was flanked by his parents at the funeral. He hugged them both and thanked them for their understanding.

Elizabeth believes their relationship was strengthened because of their willingness to stand by their son when he functioned in the role of Chadult. She even feels more confident about how he will deal with *them* when *they* age or become ill.

When Chadults find themselves in the role of caregiver to their husband's or wife's parents there is a great risk of anger and resentment.

There is an old story about a man who married his dead wife's sister so he wouldn't have to break in a new mother-in-law!

Despite the shattering of the stereotype of the daughter-in-law–mother-in-law relationship, there are still circumstances where bad feeling exists.

Sometimes that feeling starts as early as the wedding. One of the parties may have slighted the other. One of the parties may be angling for position with the son-fiancé. It takes a very wise man to balance these positions and have everyone feel comfortable.

Often when the two women get off to a bad start it takes enormous effort to bring about a friendship, and all too frequently very little energy is put into improving the relationship. Instead, hurts and slights, whether real or imagined, are allowed to fester and grow as the years go on.

Then comes that fateful day when Dad dies and Mother is in need of a support system.

Jim's mother, Elana, found herself in such a situation. After her husband's funeral she wandered aimlessly around her home trying to think about what she should do with her life now.

When her son, Jim called that evening she began to cry. His heart went out to her. Here she was alone, while his home was filled with teenaged children and activity.

"Why don't you come and stay with us for a week or so?" he asked.

"I'd love that. Can you pick me up tomorrow?"

"Sure. Right after work."

When he hung up he saw his wife, Candy, staring at him, her mouth agape with shock.

"You know she hates me!" she exclaimed. "You know I can't stomach her! How could you put us both in this position? I don't want her in my home overnight. Not even for *one* night—let alone a week!"

Her husband experienced a shocking jab of that "monkey in the middle" feeling. What in the world was he supposed to do now? He had promised his mother, and his wife would have none of it.

"Well," he said after several minutes of stormy silence, "I guess you have a right to have people in your home that you like. I'll just go over there right after work tomorrow and spend some time with her."

Candy was left fuming. She had the sinking sensation that comes with winning the battle and losing the war.

True to his word, Jim went directly to his mother's after work. He called home to let Candy know where he was. "I'm staying for dinner. See you later."

Candy hung up frozen with rage and an emotion she could not identify. It felt almost like fear. Things would no longer be as they once were. She was certain of that. With her father-in-law's death nothing would be the same.

One of Candy's close friends, Florence, happened to call her just then, and Candy was unable to conceal her emotions. They were plainly evident in her voice.

When she was through explaining what had occurred her friend asked if she wanted input. Candy admitted she certainly did need some advice.

"First of all, what in the world happened between you and your mother-in-law? She seems like a nice woman," Florence said.

"She didn't want her son to marry me," Candy replied. "She said he was too young. I resented that terribly, and I still do."

"You've been married twenty-three years and you still carry a grudge about that? He didn't listen to her, did he?"

"No. He and I wanted to get married as soon as we could. Instead of having a big wedding, we eloped. We didn't want her hassle! My parents told me to do whatever I wanted. So we just took off and got married."

"All these years and neither of you has tried to fix things between you? After all, it's your husband and her son who feels the pain. He must always be torn whenever family times come, or on holidays. Don't either of you understand that?"

"Are you saying that it's my fault?"

"No. I think somebody needed to step in years ago. Probably Jim should have put his foot down when he still had his father as an ally. Candy, you've got to do something. The woman is alone. Jim is an only child. What is he supposed to do, pretend she doesn't exist?"

Candy was taken aback. She had fully expected Florence to support her, but that was not what she was hearing. Instead, her friend seemed to be saying that things needed to change.

"I'll think about it," Candy said finally.

By the time her husband got home she had had several hours in which to think. She had looked around their large, well-furnished home. She had opened doors and closets filled with stylish clothing. She had looked at pictures of her happy, accomplished children, all smiling and knowing their college money was assured.

She had taken time to look through picture albums of vacations when she and her husband had looked at each other so lovingly. He was a good man. A tender man. A faithful man. He had given her a fine life.

In the course of a busy life, few people take time to look at or enumerate their blessings. But during the evening Candy had done exactly that. She had even taken the step of thinking what a fine man her husband was . . . and could he have been that person without the good, loving upbringing he had been given?

Candy met Jim at the door and took his hands in hers. In a timid voice she said, "I was wrong. I'm sorry."

Jim swooped her up in his arms and despite the pain he

still felt over his father's recent death, he hugged her and grinned.

"Well, we'll start working on healing the problem soon. It's funny, you know. My mother said the same thing to me when I got there. She said she was wrong. She was older and should have initiated some peacemaking a long time ago!"

He laughed then. "What if you two become good friends?"

Perhaps he didn't know it that night, but indeed he foretold what happened. The two women met for dinner. Both cried and began the process of making amends. Their relationship grew so strong that it almost equaled that of Ruth and Naomi in the Bible.

Ironically, there were times after that when Jim was not thrilled to come home and find his mother visiting. "I wanted you two to like each other but I still wanted a separate life with you," he told Candy.

She laughed. "You've heard the saying—'Be careful what you wish for. You might get it!' "

How fortunate this family was that they shared enough love to create a willingness to bring estranged parties together. And Jim was also putting in place the groundwork for his mother's later years, when she most likely would need help and a daughter-in-law who cared about her.

Sometimes Chadults find themselves in the situation of having an abundance of blessings: two sets of parents who are both in need of help!

Iris and Edward were one such couple. Their parents were nearing eighty. Up until recently all four of the older people had functioned well on their own. While neither mother had ever learned to drive, the fathers were still driving and their health had been relatively sound.

Within a month Iris's mother suffered a stroke and Edward's father had a heart attack and died.

Iris and Edward were so conflicted they didn't know where to run first. Both worked in professional capacities that left them little free time to spend on family matters.

When the time came for Iris's mother to leave the hospital, Iris and Edward looked at each other in dismay.

What were they going to do? Iris's father was simply too old to be caring for her mother on a full-time basis. Edward's mother was finding it painful to live alone, having been dependent on her husband for her physical needs and emotional support since their marriage fifty-odd years earlier.

As it happened, Iris and Edward had accumulated a great deal of money. Their house was quite large and their children were no longer living at home. They decided that the best use of space and time and money was to have their home divided into three units. Theirs, of course, would remain the largest. They would provide enough room for Edward's mother to have her own bedroom–sitting room and a small kitchen. They would also provide an apartment with bedroom, living room, and kitchen for Iris's parents.

They discussed what they planned to do with all three aging parents and were surprised at how gratefully the parents received their proposal.

Although it took the builder about a month to complete the project, once it was done and everyone was in place things fell together well.

Iris and Edward called a family meeting. They told their parents they still planned to live their busy lives. They established a night when they hoped all five of them could have dinner together. They suggested that the other three might want to make some arrangements of their own. Since the in-laws had always gotten on fairly well these arrangements were soon incorporated.

In addition to their live-in housekeeper, Iris and Edward hired an aide who assisted Iris's mother in her stroke recovery work and drove her to therapy sessions.

Iris and Edward still felt that their home was their own because they had arranged the remodeling for maximum privacy. At the same time, they had found the simplest, most time-efficient way of staying in close contact with all the parents.

To say everyone lived happily ever after would, of course, be a fairy tale. There were disputes and times of tension. But since the Chadults were two astute people they could almost always smell trouble brewing and frequently headed off problems before they began.

Other families face similar circumstances. There are demands from both sets of parents. Not all Chadults have the resources of Iris and Edward. They seek other solutions.

Caroline found that she was being called upon to drive two widowed mothers—hers and her husband, Leonard's—everywhere. Sarah and Sylvia would call each morning, assuming that she would be available. After a time Caroline began to feel imposed upon and was angry at being taken for granted.

"The first thing I did was insist that they sell their homes if they wanted my involvement. They both did. I then found them condominiums in the same complex. Not next door or anything like that, but in the same complex. I insisted on having a meeting so we could coordinate who needed what done and when.

"Sylvia, my mother-in-law, didn't like my tough stance. She called Leonard to complain. He told her if I'm nice enough to do her errands or take her on them then she would have to do it my way."

Caroline's own mother, Sarah, did not like the amount of time spent with her husband's mother, but Caroline soon put a stop to those complaints: "This is the way it has to be. My mother-in-law has to see her doctors and has no way to get there but me."

Caroline did all she could to reassure Sarah that she was first in her heart, but her mother was never fully reassured. "I try to do the best I can." Caroline sighs. "But I have to deal with each situation as it comes up."

She feels that neither woman realizes she has a life of her own and friends she wishes to see and things she wishes to do.

"But as long as they stick to the schedule, I guess I will have to listen to some grumbling and make the best of it. That's life."

Many experts maintain that regardless of what a woman has accomplished professionally, if she is the only female in the group of family members she will automatically be considered the prime caregiver. It does not matter if there are four retired unmarried sons. The responsibility still seems to fall on the female.

If a husband and wife can work as a team regardless of which parent or parents are involved they can save themselves much marital strife. It is necessary always to discuss plans of action before implementing them and do one another the courtesy of listening when a divergent point of view is presented.

Issues dealing with in-laws frequently dog marriages in the early days. Wise Chadults do whatever is needed to avoid such problems in their later years.

◆

Because of the large number of divorces that occur even after long marriages, a peculiar circumstance can arise.

Joellen spent forty years in a marriage before leaving her husband. When she remarried she still felt a strong loyalty to her former in-laws, the Bennetts, who had been loving and kind to her since she was a young woman.

"It's an odd situation," she says. "My new in-laws are fine people. They have been very welcoming and I appreciate that. But I still have strong feelings for my former mother-in-law and now that she is so ill I like to stop and visit.

"My husband doesn't object, thank heaven, but my new in-laws don't like it. So I go about my business and don't tell them. I'm not totally comfortable about that. But I won't drop a forty-year relationship that was so meaningful."

She adds with a smile that she never would have married her present husband if he had been the kind of man who did not understand her loyalty.

After the divorce and since her remarriage, Joellen still feels a lump in her throat when she visits Mrs. Bennett. "It's been three years now and she still has my engagement picture sitting on her dresser in its special frame!"

Joellen's former family—not her ex-husband—called her recently when their mother became ill. Mrs. Bennett needed to go to the hospital for tests, but she refused. The family asked Joellen to call because their mother would listen to her.

Of course Joellen called, and even offered to take her to the hospital. The offer was accepted immediately. Her former mother-in-law went gratefully and with apparently less fear than she had anticipated.

When Joellen left her that day the older woman kissed her and thanked her for still caring about her.

Joellen felt the tears well up in her eyes once again when she told her husband about her day.

"He gave me a big hug and told me this made him feel like I would always be there for *him* as well!"

While there are never perfect formulae for human interactions in this less-than-perfect world, if we can find that space within us that is loving and kind, it has a way of radiating to those around us and strengthening all our relationships.

There is no question that a woman like Joellen, who has the capacity to separate and properly place her disappointment on her former husband and not his family, will also, in time, be able to build a positive relationship with her new family. That is the power of love and kindness.

As we look at the different combinations that make up family in this era, there is still another group of people who need our support and kindness. We need not emulate them nor do we need to love their lifestyle. What we do need to do is learn not to judge them.

Far too many gay and lesbian couples have suffered first as individuals and then, when finally discovering a soul mate, as a unit from the negative judgments heaped upon them by society.

Some gay people have been rejected since their early years. It is necessary to remember there was a time when "coming out" was simply not done, even when people guessed a person's sexual orientation.

Many gay people now in their forties or fifties, and older, can recall the pain of the name-calling that went on during their school years. The pain has been so great for some that they have become embittered, and despite having achieved great success have never been able to let go of their anger.

Half a century ago or so it was evident to a group of teen-aged boys that there was something different about Sid. The other guys would look at girls and make off-color remarks to them. They would talk about how far they got with a girl on a Saturday night. Their hormones were starting to run strongly and conversations were mostly about girls and sex.

Sid never took part in this bantering and bragging. Instead, he would walk away.

He once tried to talk with his father about how different he felt. When Sid told him he was not interested in the kind of things the other guys wanted to talk about, his father punched him.

Their relationship withered from then on, and Sid felt isolated. He had no one to turn to.

He dreaded going to school. One of the mandatory gym requirements was swimming. The custom then was for boys to swim in the nude. The locker room was a nightmare for him. It was unsupervised and as the guys undressed they were merciless in their teasing.

Things reached a peak one day when the teasing in the locker room became intense enough for Sid to cry.

Sandor, a popular and strong young man, who empathized with the plight of this isolated boy, saw what was happening and still remembers the episode. "It was terrible. Here they all were surrounding and taunting the guy as he stood there undressed and with tears streaming down his face.

"I finally got angry enough that I just stood in front of him and told all of them if they teased Sid they would have to go through me. Then the teasing stopped."

Today, Sid is an internationally known designer whose wares are popular and whose friendship is sought after by international society. It is doubtful if he would recall the incident but it made a profound impression on his champion.

Sid is now a Chadult. His mother is dead and his father lacks for nothing financially. Every need is provided for. The only thing Sid's father does not have are his son's time and love. What the father receives is given out of duty and a sense of honor.

Sid cannot forget his father's reaction to his pain. "My father calls and needs my company but I just cannot give it to him. His rejection was so complete when I was a kid that I can't forget it."

Sid does say that the rejection did one strong, positive thing for him: it made him determined and tough. He believes that this toughness, along with his talent, is what made him rise to the top of his field.

Since more gay people are becoming open about their sexual preference, more are willing to share their particular experiences as Chadults.

The most frequently posed question seems to be "What do my parents expect from me? Where were they when I was a kid and needed their support and love? Where were they when I was being rejected? How do they expect me to respond to them when they were right alongside everyone else rejecting me?"

As we saw with Sid's situation, when the parents are older and in need of nurturing, emotional support, housing, or financial support, they are very willing to overlook the contempt and shame they felt during the gay Chadult's formative years.

While many gay people were ostracized, many others—especially half a century ago, and even more recently—forced themselves into marriage. Many had children and met their homosexual needs covertly.

Since times have become a little kinder to gays, some have left impossible marriages to share life with a partner of the same sex.

Sometimes their children simply turn their backs on these couples. But there are many who opt to maintain a relationship with their gay parent.

Bonnie was one such daughter. She had always loved her mother, Miriam, and despite all the anger and resentment poured into her ears by a raging father she could not abandon the woman who raised her.

She did, however, refuse to interact with her mother's partner, Deborah. Bonnie and her mother would meet for lunch or dinner and talk about all the things that mattered to them both, but the subject of the partner was forbidden.

Miriam, so very grateful for Bonnie's willingness to remain part of her life, did not challenge this system. Deborah, too, was understanding and made no demands.

Time went on and things remained much the same. When Bonnie got married her mother attended, unescorted. Her father had since remarried and his wife was part of the wedding party.

But then the time came when Miriam became quite ill. The doctors offered no hope of recovery and Bonnie was as upset as any daughter could be.

She came to the hospital daily, and each time Deborah would be there. As the Chadult, Bonnie was the person the doctor spoke with. Bonnie was the person asked about using life support should that become necessary.

All the while her mother's partner sat silently and was treated by the medical staff as if she were invisible.

One day Bonnie came to the hospital and saw the partner weeping and holding her mother's hand. Not an unkind person, she turned to walk out to give them their privacy, when the partner asked her to stay. Bonnie sat down in the other chair and took her mother's other hand.

Both women could see that the mother was failing and they made true eye contact for the first time. "You love her very much, don't you?" Bonnie said through her own tears.

"Yes, I do. I love her and she's my best friend."

Bonnie for the first time began to understand the level of pain the partner was experiencing. She saw that her mother was asleep and invited the partner to go down to the cafeteria to share a cup of coffee.

They each grabbed tissues from the hospital stand and left the room quietly.

That time in the cafeteria was a time of awakening for Bonnie. While she had made health-care decisions for her mother with the certainty that she was doing as her mother would have wished, she appreciated the reinforcement she received from the partner.

"Your decisions are right on target. You are doing just what your mother wanted. We talked about the 'what ifs' a lot and I'm so glad you are honoring her wishes."

Bonnie was quiet. She had never considered asking this woman for input on what her mother might have said. Yet she was sitting with the person her mother had chosen to share her life with!

As they continued to talk Bonnie began asking questions about their life together—what kinds of hobbies and vacations they enjoyed, what types of food, who did the cooking, all the routine things a daughter would ordinarily know about her mother's life even if that mother was divorced. But Bonnie had forbidden discussion about this part of her mother's life and so she knew nothing.

She was amazed to find the two women shared every interest. Bonnie herself had no one who shared *everything* with her.

One of the things that came from that coffee break was the women's plan to meet the following day and once again spend some time together. The partner was very grateful because she needed to have a friendship with Bonnie.

Like many homosexual couples, Bonnie's mother and her partner had never gotten around to dealing with legalities such as the power of attorney. The lack of this all-important document meant that the partner had no voice in how Bonnie's mother was treated medically. No one was required to listen to her suggestions. She was given no information because she had not been properly designated by the power of attorney. Consequently, Bonnie's goodwill became critical. Without that goodwill the partner was no more than a stranger to the woman she loved.

Bonnie's mother lived another six months, and they were happy months, indeed. She lived to see the two women she cared for most develop a friendship that was easy and kind.

When she died she knew her partner would not be alone. Bonnie had promised she would stay in contact and help her if it was possible.

Bonnie kept that promise and was there for the partner when she, shortly after, also became ill and died.

Sometimes gay people who are older need home care or nursing home care. It is urgent that staff be made sensitive to the gay person's sexual perference. If someone is aging or ill it is cruel to treat them with the same mockery they likely faced when they were children.

One couple had an aide come to their home who was openly contemptuous of their lifestyle. The Chadult son of one of the partners called the agency and explained the problem; another aide was sent that same day.

When Chadults help ill gay parents settle in it is wise to tell those who need to know the truth about the relationship, especially if the partner is still on the scene. An agency or a nursing home can assign appropriate people for care if they are given the information.

When gays decide to become partners and share a home and a life it is necessary for them to seek solid legal advice which will give them guidelines for making decisions and help families understand what is expected of them.

When people take on the role of caring Chadult, any number of circumstances can greet them. As the definition of "family" broadens we must learn to open our minds. It would make a fine world if we were always willing to open our hearts, and perhaps that will happen one day.

But until it does, whether we are a traditional family or a stepfamily, whether we are a close neighbor or friend, whether we have been a foster child or adopted and loved, whether we are dealing with our in-laws or our own parents, whether we are a homosexual couple or a heterosexual couple, compassion and a sense of fair play can always serve as our guide.

Thousands of years ago we were told to do unto others as we would like others to do unto us. Since all of us wish to be treated respectfully and caringly, since we want our needs met and we want our own children to love us, we must set the example by our actions and by being the kind of people who bring out these values in those around us.

Children do indeed learn what they live. When Chadults do difficult things for their parents without grumbling and anger, they are showing their own children the treatment they would like for themselves.

We were also told all those years ago to honor our fathers and our mothers. That was in a simpler time. Now it would perhaps best be said that in a world that has grown smaller and changed so dramatically in its mores, we must learn to honor everyone from child to parent.

When we learn this we bring honor to ourselves.

FOR THE BEST IN PAPERBACKS, LOOK FOR THE

In every corner of the world, on every subject under the sun, Penguin represents quality and variety—the very best in publishing today.

For complete information about books available from Penguin—including Puffins, Penguin Classics, and Arkana—and how to order them, write to us at the appropriate address below. Please note that for copyright reasons the selection of books varies from country to country.

In the United Kingdom: Please write to *Dept. JC, Penguin Books Ltd, FREEPOST, West Drayton, Middlesex UB7 0BR.*

If you have any difficulty in obtaining a title, please send your order with the correct money, plus ten percent for postage and packaging, to *P.O. Box No. 11, West Drayton, Middlesex UB7 0BR*

In the United States: Please write to *Consumer Sales, Penguin USA, P.O. Box 999, Dept. 17109, Bergenfield, New Jersey 07621-0120.* VISA and MasterCard holders call 1-800-253-6476 to order all Penguin titles

In Canada: Please write to *Penguin Books Canada Ltd, 10 Alcorn Avenue, Suite 300, Toronto, Ontario M4V 3B2*

In Australia: Please write to *Penguin Books Australia Ltd, P.O. Box 257, Ringwood, Victoria 3134*

In New Zealand: Please write to *Penguin Books (NZ) Ltd, Private Bag 102902, North Shore Mail Centre, Auckland 10*

In India: Please write to *Penguin Books India Pvt Ltd, 706 Eros Apartments, 56 Nehru Place, New Delhi 110 019*

In the Netherlands: Please write to *Penguin Books Netherlands bv, Postbus 3507, NL-1001 AH Amsterdam*

In Germany: Please write to *Penguin Books Deutschland GmbH, Metzlerstrasse 26, 60594 Frankfurt am Main*

In Spain: Please write to *Penguin Books S. A., Bravo Murillo 19, 1° B, 28015 Madrid*

In Italy: Please write to *Penguin Italia s.r.l., Via Felice Casati 20, I-20124 Milano*

In France: Please write to *Penguin France S. A., 17 rue Lejeune, F–31000 Toulouse*

In Japan: Please write to *Penguin Books Japan, Ishikiribashi Building, 2–5–4, Suido, Bunkyo-ku, Tokyo 112*

In Greece: Please write to *Penguin Hellas Ltd, Dimocritou 3, GR–106 71 Athens*

In South Africa: Please write to *Longman Penguin Southern Africa (Pty) Ltd, Private Bag X08, Bertsham 2013*